Potty Training for Boys in 3 Days

Guide to Diaper-Free, Stress-Free Toilet Training for Your Toddler (2022 for Beginners)

Adele Nicholls

Table of Contents

CHAPTER 1

    BACKGROUND IN 1

CHAPITRE 2

    ARE YOU TOO YOUNG? ARE YOU OLD ENOUGH? 17

CHAPITRE 3:

    HOW TO DETERMINE THE BEST TIME TO BEGIN 21

CHAPITRE 4

    MAKE YOURSELF READY 26

CHAPITRE 5

    THE CHILD'S PREPARATION 35

CHAPITRE 6

    CALENDAR FOR POTTY-TRAINING..43

CHAPTER 7

    EQUIPMENT ARSENAL 47

CHAPTER 8

    THREE-DAY POTTY-TRAINING METHOD 53

CHAPITRE 9

    WHEN NOTHING ELSE WORKS 63

CHAPTER 11

    SPECIALITIES OF BOY POTTY TRAINING 74

CHAPITRE 12

    REWARDS AND CELEBRATION 78

CHAPITRE 13

    REPEAT EAT, PLAY, POOP 81

CHAPITRE 14

    MANAGING ACCIDENTS 84

CHAPTER 15 BONUS

    41 MODERN PARENTING SOLUTIONS AND TIPS 87

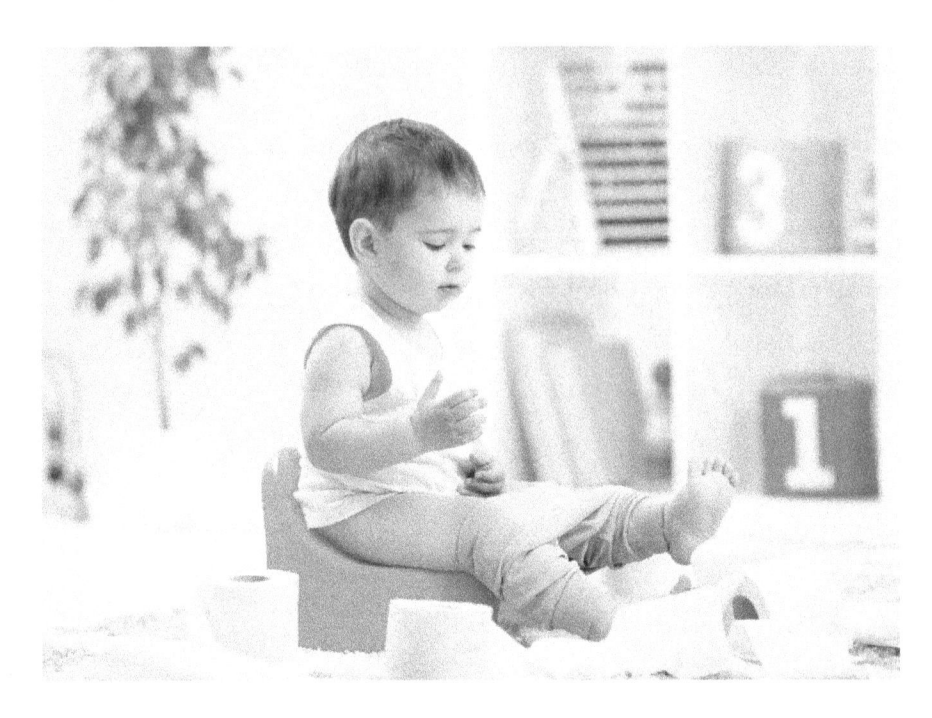

Having children is an amazing experience for parents all around the world. Children provide some lovely memories, but one of the more difficult memories is changing soiled diapers.

No parent like this duty, and figuring out how to educate your child to use the potty can be challenging, especially if putting a system in place has not been at the top of your priority list.

In this book, we will look at some of the most effective toilet training strategies for your kid to guarantee that he understands everything and uses the potty. Most parents are unclear about how to teach their children to use the potty and when to start potty training. There are several potty-training options available, and it is critical to select the best one for your child. Whether or whether he learns will be determined by his desire and readiness to cooperate.

Don't start potty training too soon. According to studies, when parents start potty training their children too soon, it takes them longer to learn.

master the ability So, when your child is ready to begin training, you will have success.

The first step is to use the information in this book to determine whether your child is ready to be potty trained. Concentrate on the plans when he is ready. Maintain a simple schedule for your child. If he has recently started daycare or has a younger brother or sister, he may be less receptive to change. Wait until he is more open to change before beginning toilet training.

Looking for signs of readiness is one approach to determining when your toddler is ready to be toilet trained. These symptoms include hunching and grunting, as well as remaining dry for three hours or more. When you understand and recognize these common signs of potty-training readiness, you can decide when to start preparing your child to use the potty. Potty train your child only when he is ready!

Please keep this in mind: No child should be potty trained until he or she is ready. In this case, your youngster has complete control. He can be gently coaxed, but not coerced, into using the restroom. Toilet training requires patience, calm, and teaching your youngster to figure things out on his or her own.

CHAPTER I

BACKGROUND IN

"Why to bother potty training?" some parents wonder. "Don't things just fall into place?" Or they believe that if a youngster is exposed to the routine of potty training early enough, he will learn to go to the toilet on his own. That, however, is not the case.

Many people believe that older children (four years and more) potty train faster than younger children (one to three years). Some of the assumptions that sometimes arise from the medical profession, modern-daycare, or the community are as follows:

Children cannot successfully toilet train until the "myelination of the sphincters" occurs, and attempts to toilet train them before this time will be futile.

Every toddler ultimately learns to use the toilet - have you ever seen an adult who isn't toilet trained?

Children as young as four years old can begin to prepare for school; no child in secondary school is in diapers.

It is true that some infants "prepare themselves." These are children that grow up in homes where parents make potty or toilet facilities available to their children from birth, without labeling it "training."

In any case, if we're talking about a one-and-a-half to a three-year-old child who isn't yet potty-trained, he isn't ready.

prepared to train himself Unfortunately, some parents are confined by work or social settings and are unable to play an active role in assisting their child in becoming potty trained, even after determining what their child needs.

Potty training is a vital activity for preparing a child's body to reap the benefits of what is frequently referred to as man's most important innovation - indoor plumbing/sanitation. One of the most basic prerequisites for long-term health is the ability to use the restroom.

Your child's physical ability to be potty trained fall into place simply; nevertheless, as with other areas where the body meets hardware, critical training is required. We get excited about our baby's first word, first tooth, and first steps (tears of joy!), but we cringe at the prospect of cleaning up the messes required for our child to learn self-toileting. Diapers, pull-ups, padded trousers, and other similar items keep pee and poop out of sight for an extended period.

However, if we reconsider potty training, we will discover that it is both a means to an end and an opportunity to bond with our child. Its benefits extend far beyond the toilet seat.

Potty training in different countries

While we struggle to juggle work and parenthood, we avoid discussing potty training with our children since the topic is considered disgusting or unsavory. But that hasn't always been the case with our global neighbors, and it still isn't today.

Moms from other parts of the world may be surprised by the commotion surrounding potty training. They appear to know when to potty train intuitively since they frequently keep their toddlers close to their bodies.

These cues are tough to ignore when holding your child on your side. It's much simpler to miss them if they're fifteen feet away on a mat. African and Asian mothers carry their children throughout the day, so they instinctively know when it is time to take their newborn children away from them to relieve themselves.

In a big section of Europe, parents claim that their infants send indications when they need to go, thus they don't wear diapers all day. The potty is available in Germany; however, toddlers are allowed to use it at their speed. In France, no child begins school in diapers, and children aged one to three years are not authorized to attend playgroups in diapers.

Parents in China and India start potty training their children at a young age.

When babies are a year old, their parents or caregivers usually place them over the potty after the main meal and make a suggestive "shush" sound for urinating or an "uh, uh" sound to assist an infant in pooping.

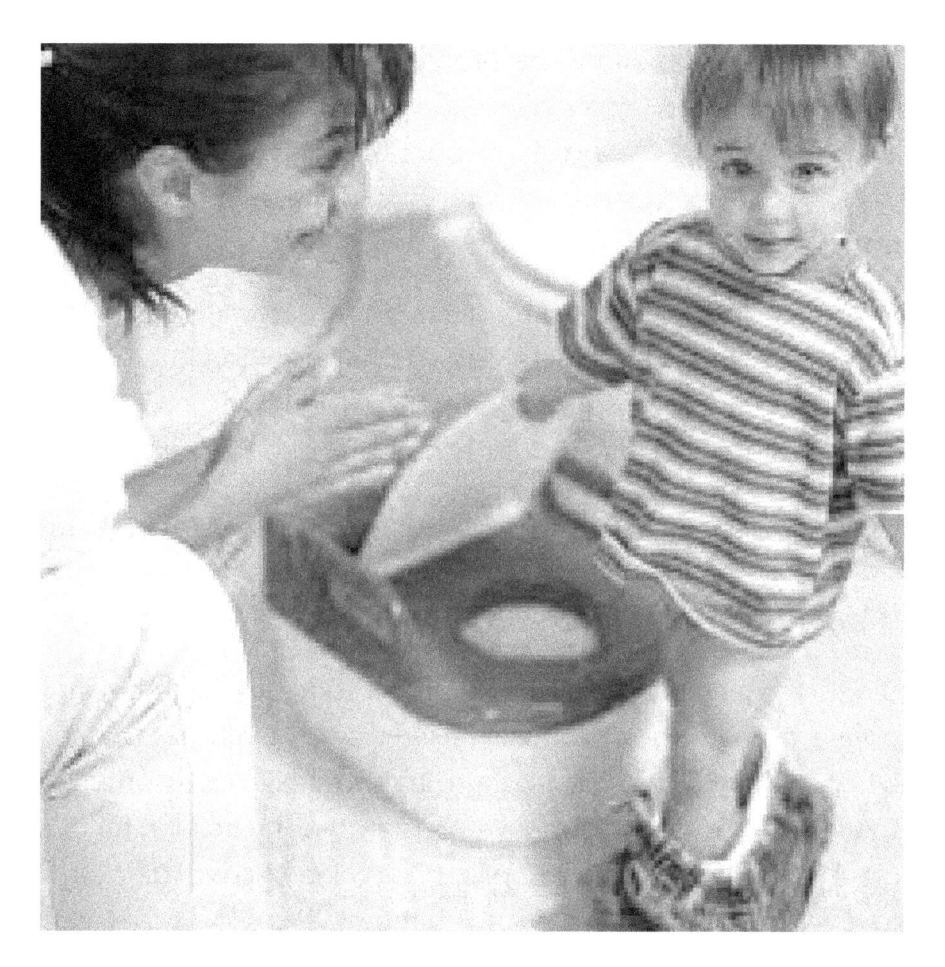

This takes some time, but once the kids get the hang of it, they do both without fail. In China, small children frequently wear pants with a rear split through which they can discharge themselves.

Parents in countries where parents keep their very young toddlers close to them learn to read their child's signs. The youngster adjusts, but the parent is the one who is best prepared. Parents that use "no diaper" tactics from birth are dedicated, and it's something that any parents could do if they chose to.

Because bowel motions are strongly associated with health and well-being in Japan, discussions about potty training are prevalent. They even have cartoons and children's books to teach both parents and children the benefits of using the potty.

One thing that all of these mothers have in common is that they prefer to start potty training early rather than later. This is significant because they prefer terrycloth or bird eye cotton diapers to super-absorbent disposables. The youngster expresses pain in dirty or wet diapers more quickly, which acts as a signal to begin toilet training.

The Evolution of Potty Training

Diaper material has traditionally been a deciding element in potty training. When diapers were made of cloth or cotton wool, getting children out of them immediately was essential. There was no debate about when to start potty training for a pioneer mother with endless piles of clothing and wet diapers to dry (sometimes without washing them). It was ideal to start teaching toddlers to use the toilet as soon as possible. This occasionally led to extreme measures such as bowel purges and suppositories.

In the 1950s, washing machines helped relieve moms' burdens.

However, because mothers were still wearing cloth diapers, they were aware of their child's timetables and signals and would place them on the potty when the child was expected to go. The child would then associate his gestures with being made to use the potty. It was common for youngsters to be potty trained by the age of 18 months.

Disposable diapers were much more inexpensive in the 1980s. Parents could use cloth diapers or disposable diapers.

Parents were no longer as eager to potty train their toddlers at a young age.

This was around the time that doctor Dr. T. Brazelton Berry and the American Academy of Pediatrics advocated for a potty-training method as a response to the very harsh schedules used in the previous century. Instead of rushing, parents were advised to wait until the youngster could express his requirements. The emphasis gradually shifted from the demands of the parents to the needs of the child.

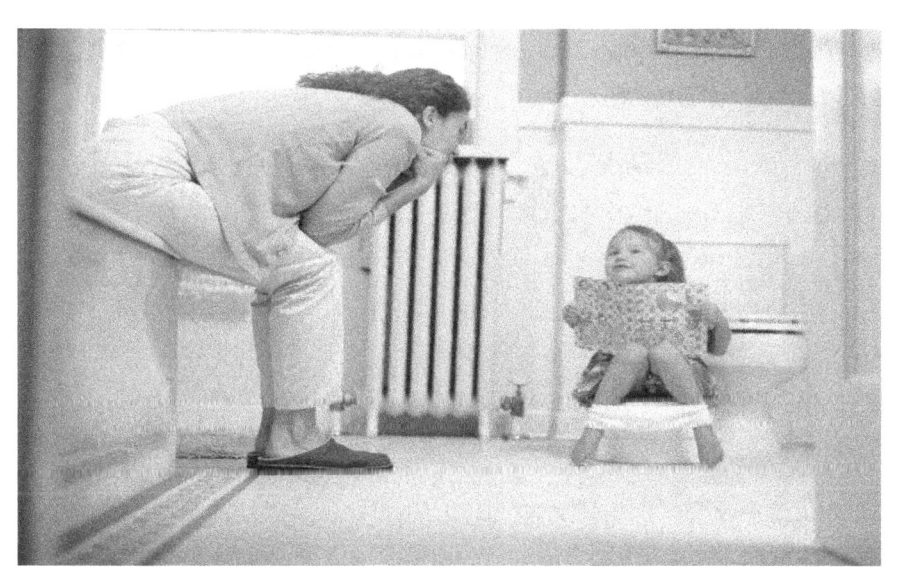

The pendulum has now entirely swung away from early potty training. Disposable diapers are no longer an option; they are the norm. With more women working outside the home and diapers becoming more affordable, we aren't compelled to potty train our children just to reduce our workload. Potty training is optional. We now see no harm in children using diapers well into their toddler years.

Potty training children under one-year-old has been abandoned in Western countries such as Australia, the United States, the United Kingdom, and many European countries. It is now considered acceptable to delay potty training until a child is three years old.

In any event, delayed potty training causes a slower development of

additional learning talents of a youngster the constant advice of modern-day childcare specialists to "wait until the toddler is ready" can be confusing.

be reckless since most parents are ill-equipped to determine when their child is ready.

Many parents rely on rewards rather than educating their children to use the restroom freely. This may work for some, but it frequently results in tense, out-of-control bartering between parent and child, especially with youngsters who have discovered how to express their disobedience in words or who refuse to go along when rewards are no longer available. Furthermore, bartering is completely ineffective.

Others view potty training as a mystery, with no framework and little attention to the toddler's cues. The disadvantage is that, while this appears to be training, it will take longer because both parent and child are dissatisfied when there does not appear to be any long-term improvement with this strategy.

Finally, some people forgo developing potty skills and instead rely on commercial products to meet their potty demands. Who wouldn't think that it's easier to put a disposable diaper on a child than it is to teach him?

If anyone has missed the point about who is driving this change in potty training, it is the diaper manufacturers.

They have gained by delaying diaper use in older children, even producing larger-sized diapers for youngsters as young as four and five years old. As a result, the average potty-training age in America has now risen to 30 months (but it can reach 60 months)!

Because disposables keep moisture away from the skin, there is less incentive for both parents and children to start potty training.

Infants and small children do not understand what it is like to be wet.

According to research, approximately 90 percent of American children wear disposables, and only approximately 10 percent are potty trained by a year and a half, even though 95 percent of children were potty trained by a year and a half not long ago, even without the unforgiving potty-training techniques of the mid-1900s.

When should today's youngsters be potty trained?

Half of all children worldwide are potty trained by the age of one year, with some even by six months. The great majority of children worldwide are potty trained by the age of two.

Most boys in the United States are not potty trained until they are 35 to 39 months old (about three years old).

This concerning trend has not gone ignored. Child healthcare services have issued wide assessments and recommendations on how to change this situation around. However, while first-world countries address the issue of delayed toilet training, the trend of giving the practice of early potty training is gaining popularity among China's white-collar class and other newly developing nations.

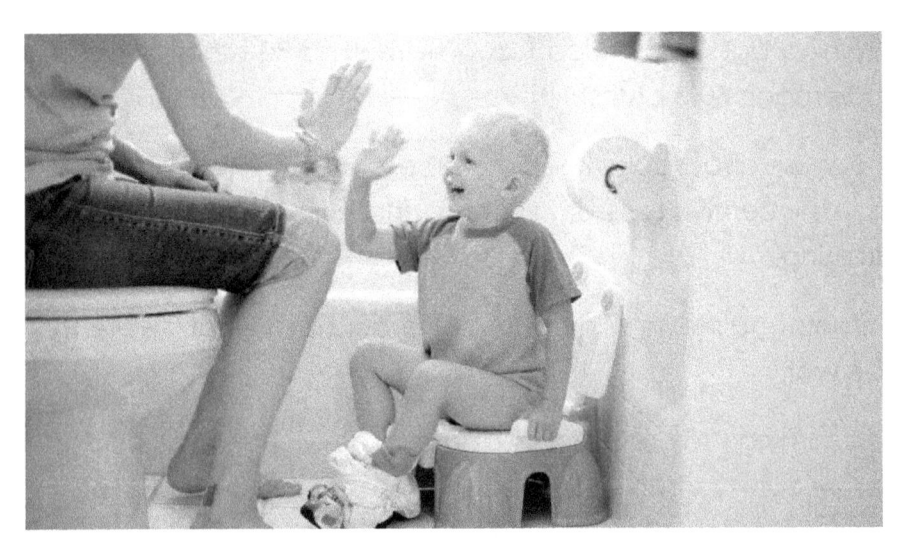

It is still typical in Hong Kong to try to avoid the long-term usage of diapers. Despite all of its achievements, individuals in China prefer to avoid using diapers since they are still quite expensive. However, as more Chinese people become wealthy, there is a greater need for diapers.

Instead of thinking it's strange that a school-age kid isn't yet potty-trained, people now frown on parents who train their children.

child younger than two years old One woman who began toilet training her child before he was two revealed that people chastised her for doing so, stating it was "too soon."

Controlling bodily excretion is an important aspect of human development. It is the first form of self-control that small toddlers develop. Today, toddlers learn to use complex technological devices at ages when they had previously achieved continence.

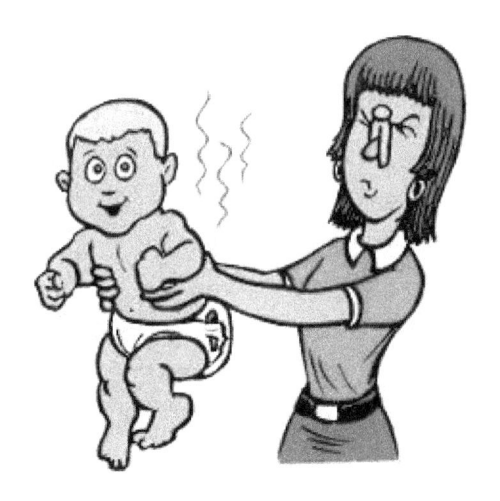

Potty Training to Meet Today's Demands

Lots of affection is required for a successful potty-training strategy. The distinction between severe and healthy treatments is determined by love. The greatest tactics are ones that encourage, rather than compel, potty training while also being stern enough to leave a mark on a child's muscle memory.

We shall take some time to rediscover what mothers all across the world have known since the beginning. We'll mix the best of what we've learned from many sources to discover how we may best teach our children.

Early toilet training motivations

Parents in Japan are encouraged to potty train their children as early as possible to reduce the load on others, such as friends, instructors, or childcare providers. The more children that come to class in diapers, the less time there is for instruction.

Preschool teachers who have inexperienced three-year-old's in their classes waste time changing diapers instead of teaching. This is problematic, especially for educators who come from countries where toddlers are not allowed to start nursery or preschool until they are potty trained. "I believe it's foolish not to try to get toddlers out of diapers by three years of age," one instructor said.

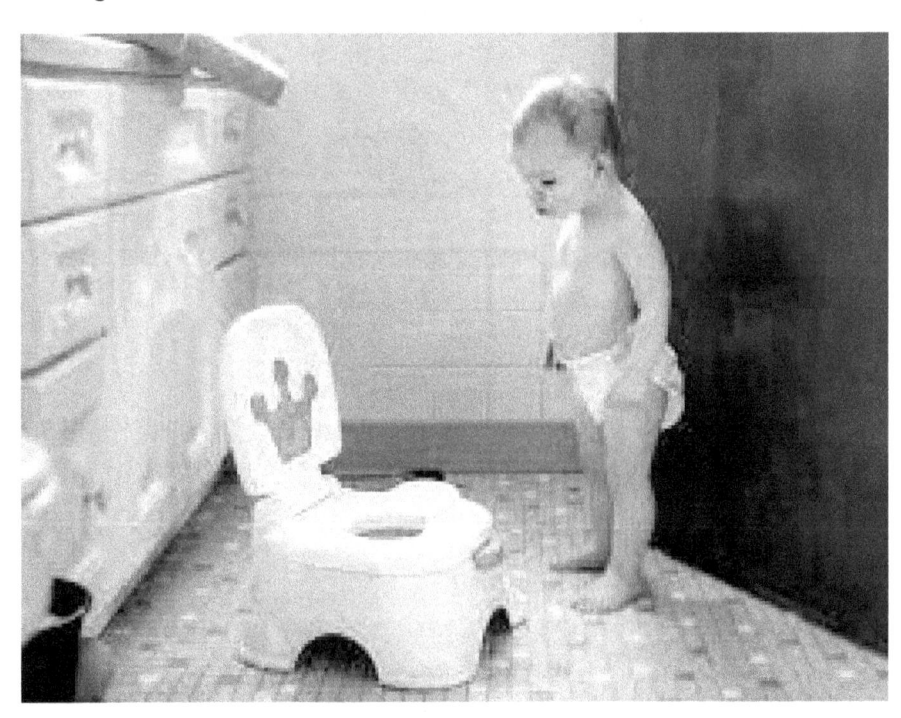

At the same time, children who have experienced basic potty training at home can serve as supportive role models for their classmates.

Someone may be unsure how to assist oneself When two, three, and four-year-olds observe others using the toilet, they swiftly learn. Their

It makes a difference to follow a consistent pattern.

Clean and sterile Parents who start toilet training their children between the ages of one and three find it cleaner, less expensive, and more convenient.

and well-timed for the child's autonomy and independent development They don't give it much thought; they simply begin potty-training when they notice that their children are ready. They don't begin with the expectation that it will be a difficult task; instead, they just lead the way in starting and supporting their child.

They will never have to pick up after their toddlers again.

These parents believe that by keeping children in diapers for longer periods, Western culture has regressed. They feel that a toddler requires consistent close encouragement and training for sterile potty training to occur without the usage of diapers. Potty training a toddler at a young age is undeniably cleaner and more pleasant.

Environmentally friendly

There's also little debate about what's better for the environment: weaning your child from diapers early saves a lot of garbage. Cloth diapers pollute the environment less than disposable diapers. Every day, a typical child gets changed six to eight times. That equates to approximately 3000 disposable diapers for each child every year!

Disposable diapers generate a large amount of waste because they are sometimes thrown in household recycling bins; their waste contaminates the other post-consumer paper, rendering it inappropriate for reuse. Disposable diapers are also a litter problem on beaches and in areas with few or no public garbage cans.

Less expensive, less financial strain

Parents who can afford disposables tend to toilet train later, whereas budget-conscious parents tend to train earlier. Regardless of financial means, parents who plan ahead of time reap the distinct benefit of having a potty-trained child sooner than those who rely solely on diapers.

More parental focus on the child

Potty training allows parents to give their children more attention and support as they strive toward the end goal.

While full-time homemakers are in the best position to toilet-train their children, working mothers have an added incentive to provide the necessary attention and assistance.

Working mothers who choose to potty train their children early benefit from lower upkeep and other benefits. Such who do not begin training as soon as possible lose those benefits.

This training also provides an opportunity for you to bond with your child. Furthermore, we can see that it has a favorable impact on family ties.

It Aids a toddler's independence and self-sufficiency.

Although many parents are concerned about their children's intellectual development, they are less concerned about their toddlers

Many mothers have observed a correlation between the self-control developed during potty training and the overall advancement of their children while wearing diapers.

child.

Reduces potential health issues

There are numerous other advantages to potty training.

These include lowering the risk of lower urinary tract disease and bladder rupture, as well as chronic constipation and colon problems.

What happens to individuals who do not potty train at a young age?

Unnecessary humiliation

There is no clear guideline for when to quit using diapers.

Health issues

Potty training at a later age might be difficult.

A healthy approach

What we're aiming for is a healthy potty-training strategy that encompasses all of the circumstances needed for proper training

This includes training for parents, responding to children's needs, preparing the body and brain, and recognizing recurring signals. Now it's a matter of bringing the difficulties to light so that parents can recognize that potty training should begin between the ages of one and three.

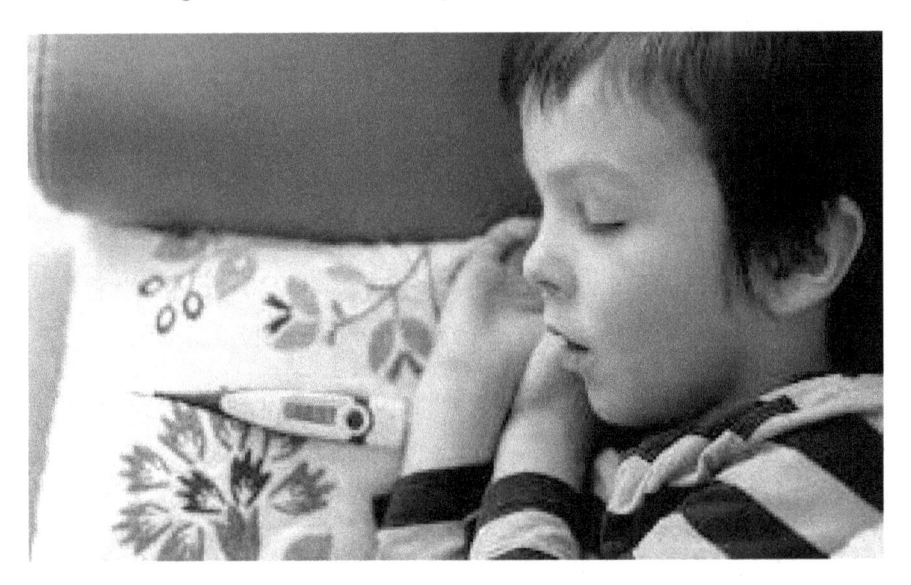

Unlike training during the "terrible twos," when youngsters announce their independence and rebel, this can be a smooth and flawless procedure.

Potty training can be used as an act of defiance.

The Three-Day Method's Effectiveness

Potty training in a short period works successfully for many parents, while it is not currently the standard. The Three-Day Method described in this book has assisted numerous youngsters in making the crucial transition away from diapers. It has also aided many parents in becoming more acquainted with their children outside of the confines of their routines and responsibilities.

Using this or other training methods does not guarantee that your child will be fully potty trained in three days. Rather, your youngster will be using the potty instead of diapers in three days.

However, accidents may occur, and you'll need to build a consistent potty habit - helping your child use the potty freely, showing him how to pull his pants down, flush the potty, and wash his hands - until one day he's doing it without accidents!

It may appear like teaching a youngster to use the potty in three days is too wonderful to be true. However, it only takes three days for two-year-old toddlers to learn the fundamentals of potty training. A few youngsters learn it faster, especially if their parents are persistent and structured before the "Three Days."

Potty training is more complicated than simply pulling off your toddler's diaper and giving him or her some instructions, but despite the effort, you will soon appreciate the sweet success of having your child potty trained.

CHAPITRE 2

ARE YOU TOO YOUNG? ARE YOU OLD ENOUGH?

Potty training is recommended for children aged one to three years.

Potty training is a significant developmental milestone for children. Most children are ready to begin potty training between the ages of one and one-and-a-half years. Regardless, some children will show evidence of being prepared earlier or later than expected. Every child is unique and will have a different experience.

In contrast to the popular belief that a toddler cannot control his pee and poop until he is older, research on child development shows that the sphincter muscles that control bladder and bowel movements begin developing while the child is in utero and reach FULL maturity between the ages of 12 months and three years. This is the time to finish, not start, toilet training.

When parents wait until these muscles have fully developed before starting potty training, the muscles have been harmed.

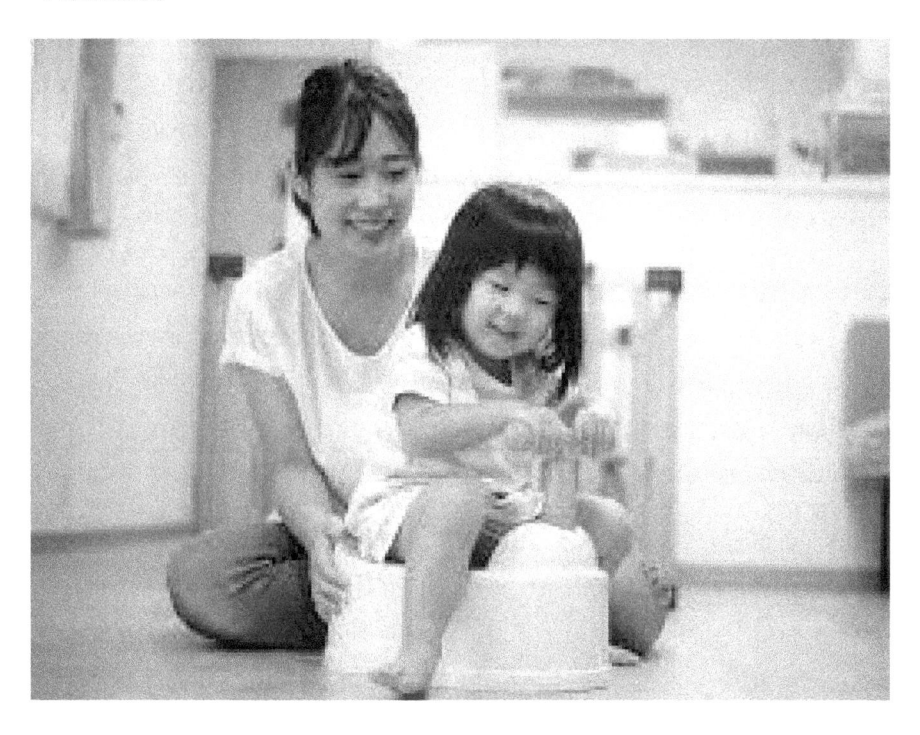

diminished by the lack of regular use that occurs when a youngster learns toilet control It is our responsibility as parents to respond to signals of readiness and provide the chance for potty training as soon as possible.

At that age, "a lot of tiny children begin to display an enthusiasm for the potty chair or toilet," you may start seeing readiness signals. Pediatricians believe that most toddlers have a "window" when they are easiest to potty train.

This window is usually around two to two-and-a-half years of age for girls, and around two-and-a-half to three years of age for males, after which time children can establish a long-term habit of diaper use or just refuse potty training.

Inexperienced parents may believe that the earlier a toddler becomes acquainted with the potty, the longer the real potty training will take, but this is not true. Children who begin training between the ages of 19 months and two years have the best outcomes. Typically, these children are out of diapers by the age of 25 months.

Some children are trained easily when their parents wait until they are about two and three years old, but others take longer than those in the 19-month to two-year timeframe, partially because their toilet training coincides with the "terrible twos" era.

If you notice that your child is not ready to begin potty training, don't push him. There could be a variety of factors going on that are causing him concern or reluctance. When your toddler expresses significant reluctance to potty training, you should delay potty training for about a month and then try to approach potty training again without publicizing it ahead of time.

In any instance, they will be effective as long as the child is willing and the parents put in the effort.

There is no set age for beginning potty training.

The transition from diapers to underwear will go much more smoothly if you search for evidence of the child's readiness rather than being focused on starting at a specific age.

Physical and mental readiness is required for successful potty training. It is our responsibility as parents to recognize this and not load a child with a burden he is not prepared for.

CHAPITRE 3:

HOW TO DETERMINE THE BEST TIME TO BEGIN

Do you remember how exciting it was to learn to ride a bike and be able to leave the tricycle behind? That provides you a sense of how it feels for a child to go from diapers to using the potty. There may be times when it appears as if nothing will ever work, but when it does, it is thrilling.

Every child will demonstrate readiness at a different period than others within the window of time that seems to be optimum for potty training. Younger siblings may rush to the potty chair to imitate an older sibling, or a youngster may be delayed because there is an unhappy moment in the family around the time, he would ordinarily be ready. The most important thing, however, is that you as a parent can recognize when your child is READY.

Many parents have expressed their inability to determine when their child is ready for potty training on multiple occasions. Here are some common warning indicators to check for:

The child appears to be interested in the toilet or potty chair.

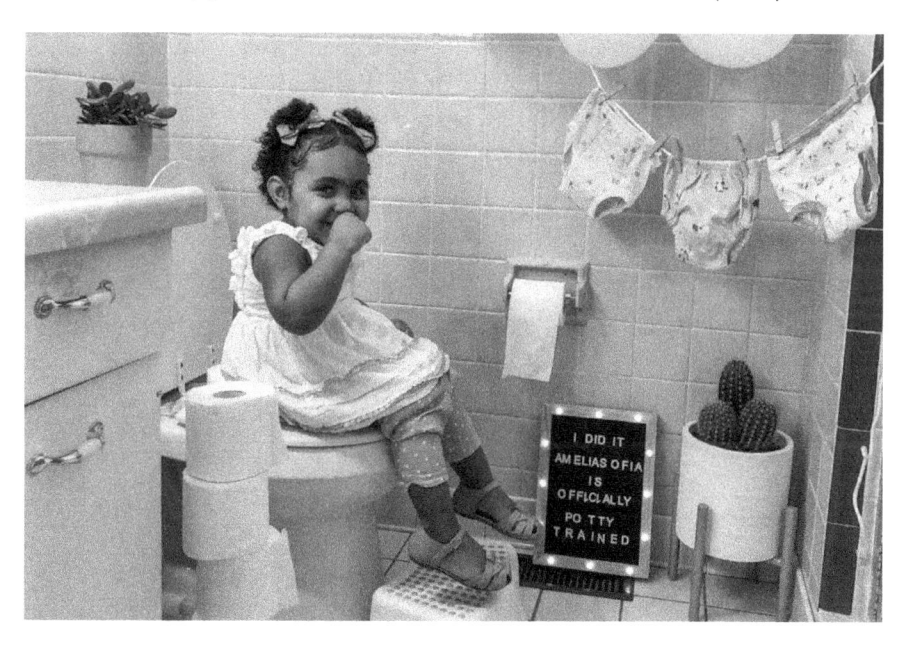

Watching others use the bathroom may encourage the youngster (this may feel uncomfortable and unpleasant at first, but it is a good way to introduce things).

The child may observe you using the toilet and ask questions about the toilet or sitting on the potty.

When another person is using the toilet, the child becomes excited.

Apart from displaying any interest in the toilet, global readiness skills are required.

Capable of walking and sitting without assistance for short periods

Can sit on and get out of a toilet seat

Can support himself on his feet and push when he has a bowel movement

Around the house, he imitates his parents.

Begins to show an interest in pleasing parents or caretakers.

Can put things back where they belong

Has a better awareness of where things go in the house and are more self-sufficient when it comes to completing responsibilities.

Desires to be self-sufficient

It can keep diapers dry for up to two hours.

This implies that he is prepared to hold urine in his bladder.

You must be able to sleep without a cup or glass.

Even if the bowel cycle is not yet regular, the individual has normal and formed bowel motions.

Can express his or her desires

Not necessarily with words, but with body movements, looks, hand gestures, or other motions

Can understand and obey simple instructions like "Give the ball to Daddy."

Understands terms related to toileting

When he poops or pees in his diaper or is about to, he tells you (or gives strong signals).

Parents must understand how their child communicates. It could start with physical discomfort, then wriggles and squirms, then small sounds and words, which is pre-language.

Is bothered by damp or soiled diapers

Complains about damp or filthy diapers, or acts out by ripping his diaper off and peeing on the floor

This means his or her diaper is damp or soiled. When a toddler is uncomfortable or embarrassed with having a wet diaper, he is ready for potty training.

When his diaper is dirty, he may request that it be changed or even attempt to remove the poop from his diaper.

Looks down at his diaper before peeing to become conscious that it will be wet.

Request to wear garments or not use a diaper.

He or she may even be able to pull down and draw up his or her pants with little assistance.

Not all of these indicators will be present when your kid is ready for potty training. Most children demonstrate preparedness with only a few of these indicators, but a general pattern of these indicators will tell you it's a perfect time to start.

Again, if your child has recently experienced or will soon experience a significant shift, for example, moving to a new home or the arrival of another sibling, it is advisable to wait a short time before fully preparing. A small child who resists potty training now will be much more ready in a month.

Try not to feel obligated to start before your youngster indicates readiness.

Also, don't be swayed by anyone, no matter who they are.

Parents, in-laws, friends, relatives, or co-workers are all examples of relatives. It will not work if your child is not ready to potty train.

Half-measures simply prolong the process of potty training, making it disappointing rather than gratifying. Even as adults, we recognised that our digestive system and elimination can change depending on our emotions and moods, and a child is no exception. When the time comes, you can utilize the three-day approach to train your child, and he will quickly learn how to use the potty chair.

CHAPITRE 4

MAKE YOURSELF READY

Gardening and cookery show on television have a way of making what they do appear simple enough for us to replicate. The hues are enticing; everyone is rosy-cheeked and healthy, and entirely at ease with the culinary or gardening expert.

The movements are so fluid; the culinary professional pulls carrots from the perfect garden, whips up a carrot smoothie, and hands it to a waiting toddler, who eats it and smiles! It appears to be quite straightforward. We conclude that we require such a garden, as well as the same nutritious food.

We imagine that we could grow the same veggies and make the same nutritious smoothies as seen on television. So, we go to the hardware store, buy some equipment, and begin digging a garden plot. It doesn't take long for us to discover that this endeavor isn't going to be as straightforward as it appears. We lose interest and give up after a short period of hard labor with no instant reward.

When it comes to potty training, many parents are like that. They look forward to putting training as a kind of "D-day" in their child's growth. The end of the diaper change is near! Unfortunately, many of these parents are unwilling to consider the amount of effort required to potty train their children. Who wants to consider that?

In actuality, anything that will offer tremendous enjoyment or value, in the end, must be approached with care and a certain degree of effort. We must be prepared and willing to put in some effort to educate our child the fundamentals of potty training. Some toddlers catch it within a few days. Some take a little longer than others. We should be prepared to work with it for however long it takes. I promise it will be worth it in the end, and it won't take as long as you think.

Here's a bad way to start toilet training, but it occurs all the time: we start potty training because we find out another child is on the way. Family and friends come from all over to shower us with love and concern, and while they're at it, they also shower us with advice. The fact that their children can occasionally be little terrors rather than the little angels they portray is a point that is sometimes overlooked in the advice.

When we learn that another child is on the way, we begin to consider moving our elder child out of diapers as soon as possible. We begin to anticipate the allotted hour with trepidation. We're prepared and have all of the essential equipment. We have a mental vision of how potty training should go: a little drama, maybe some silliness, but most importantly, a neat, joyful ending.

We bring out the toilet chair on the scheduled day, almost expecting our youngster to cheer and smile when he sees it. When he refuses to use the potty chair, pushes it away, or tears when he sees it, we are deeply disappointed. "What went wrong?" we wonder.

When the dust settles and we've recovered a little from the fact that our potty-training effort was a failure despite our best efforts, we suddenly realize that we overlooked the most critical factor.

That has to be taken into account: the child's preparedness to be potty trained.

Potty training isn't a one-time event like going camping, repainting the kitchen, or finishing some chore that someone else was expected to do. The first individuals who need to be prepared for the three days of potty training are us, the parents, and one of the things we need to do is figure out how to recognize the symptoms that our kid is ready to defecate or pee.

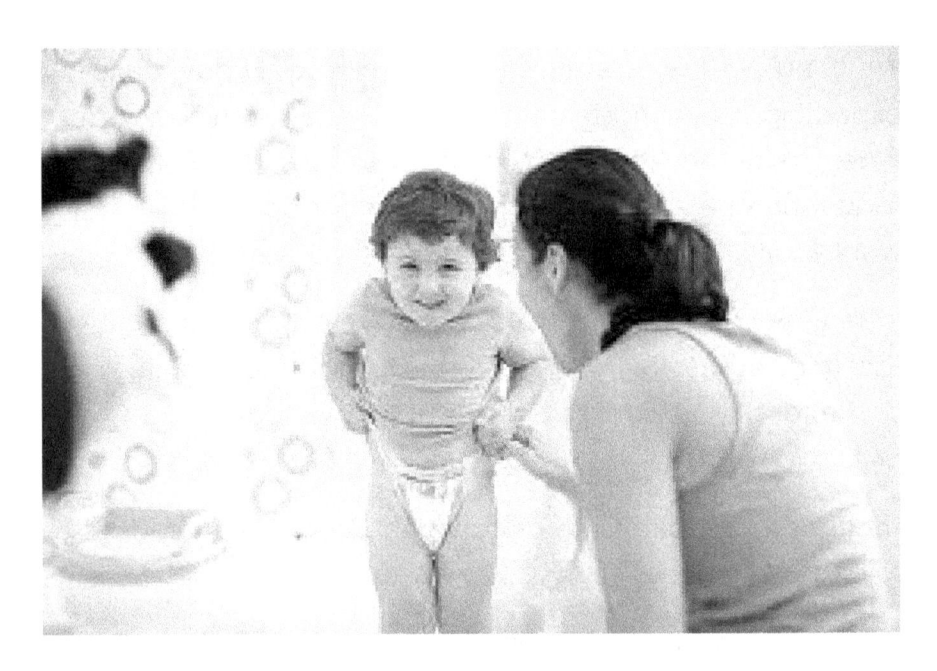

Potty training may only take three days, but we must be committed to it for much longer. Potty training is part of our commitment to the small person we brought into the world.

You may relax when you consider potty training as a crucial component of your child's overall well-being, much like eating or sleeping. You can train your youngster in a relaxed manner. You don't have to be concerned. You may make your child's transition from diapers to the potty smoother by being casual. You can unwind once you've completed the following tasks:

Allow yourself to let go of your desires.

Stop comparing the child you are potty training to other children, including your own.

Understand how your toddler's body and mind work.

Recognize readiness indicators

Determine when and how to start potty training.

Learn how to talk about potty training with your child.

Understand what concerns and difficulties to expect.

Consider how you were trained to use the toilet.

Participate in all aspects of your child's education.

Before bringing out the potty chair, it is beneficial if you have already established a routine with your child that includes other areas of learning. When your child already has a daily routine, you may include the potty into it without it being a drastic shift that may frighten rather than entice him.

Children must still understand what is expected of them. If your child starts moving toward potty training naturally or because he senses it is something you want from him, you can be a tremendous help by providing advice and applauding his efforts, but remember not to push him beyond his preparedness.

Some children are truly ready for potty training much sooner than others, so you aren't "pushing" your child if you aren't encountering any resistance. However, if there is resistance, it should be taken as a warning that the youngster is not ready. At the same time, children enjoy learning how adults do things, so don't deny them the opportunity if they are ready.

Start potty training when both you and your child are ready.

Your child may be ready for potty training, but are you? Do you already have more on your plate than you can handle?

Have you had a new child recently? When you realize that your child is ready, consider if you can commit the entire three days to teaching your child how to use the potty. When you decide on the best moment to implement the three-day plan, you should be as prepared as your kid.

Set aside all of your typical activities for three days.

Try not to schedule potty training around a time when you have a lot on your plate, such as when you are moving or expecting another kid. It's preferable to wait until things have settled down and you have a regular schedule so that you and your child can deal with setbacks and surprises with enthusiasm and joy.

During those three days, organize stand-ins or substitute aid for day-to-day activities. However, make sure to inform any relatives or friends that come to help you that you won't be able to visit and chat with them as usual because you need to focus on the child who is being potty trained. Nothing must divert your attention.

so that you are always present when your child has to defecate or pee

Choose three days when you have no other obligations or reschedule any that you do have. A long weekend is ideal. If you have other toddlers, try to locate babysitters for them or keep them occupied with TV for the majority of the day. Prepare meals ahead of time for those three days, or have enough money set aside for take-out.

Choose your vocabulary.

Make sure that all family members, long-term childcare providers, or teachers follow the same schedule with your child and use the same terms for body parts and bathroom functions. Tell them how you're going about things and ask them to follow suit so your child doesn't get confused.

Make plans to devote your time and energy to your child.

You are ready to potty train when you are willing to devote the time and energy required to help your child through the process. Keep in mind that depending on how you read his signs and readiness, you may need to approach potty training this toddler differently than you did with your other children.

Potty training guys is not the same as potty training girls. Furthermore, how one little boy responds to the teaching will differ from another. Don't be surprised if one youngster learns to use the toilet faster than another; that's just the way it is.

When things become rough, try not to return to diapers.

Potty training is a process that will inevitably have some setbacks, and your child will eventually get over wetting himself. You must continue the procedure in normal clothing rather than resorting to training pants or pull-ups, which may confuse the child. You can wipe up the pee or clean up the excrement for as long as the procedure takes, knowing that it will eventually click with them.

Determine how your kid indicates the need to pee or poop.

React quickly if you notice signals that your child may need to use the potty, such as facial gestures, squirming, hunching down, or gripping his crotch. Help your child get familiar with these indications so that he will stop what he is doing and rush to the toilet.

Praise your youngster for informing you when he has to use the restroom.

Allow your child to flush the toilet when the time comes. Make sure he washes his hands after using the restroom.

Some parents experiment with putting their child on the potty chair whether or not they have indicated a need to go. Or they may notice that their child has bowel movements at a certain time and try to put him or her on the potty at that moment.

This strategy does not work for all children, and I do not recommend it. Genuine toilet training begins when the child learns to correlate the feeling of wanting to poop or pee with getting to the potty on time. To get the youngster to use the potty, it is better to wait until he truly needs to go.

If at all feasible, limit the number of persons involved in the actual potty training.

If your spouse or grandma assists with potty training, make sure you both use comparable language and terms to avoid confusing the child. However, ideally, the parent who has observed indicators of readiness and has developed a pattern with the kid should be the one to initiate potty training.

If you are breastfeeding, you can still toilet-train your older child if you have established a regular pattern with the new baby. Your toddler will typically be pleased to help you with the baby, but when he needs to go potty, stop feeding the infant and respond to the requirements of your toilet-training toddler.

When potty training seems especially difficult, recall the inspiring motivations for the training you're performing. You may need to tell yourself, "A few days of

Having to clean up several accidents is far preferable to dealing with stinky dirty diapers for a couple of years."

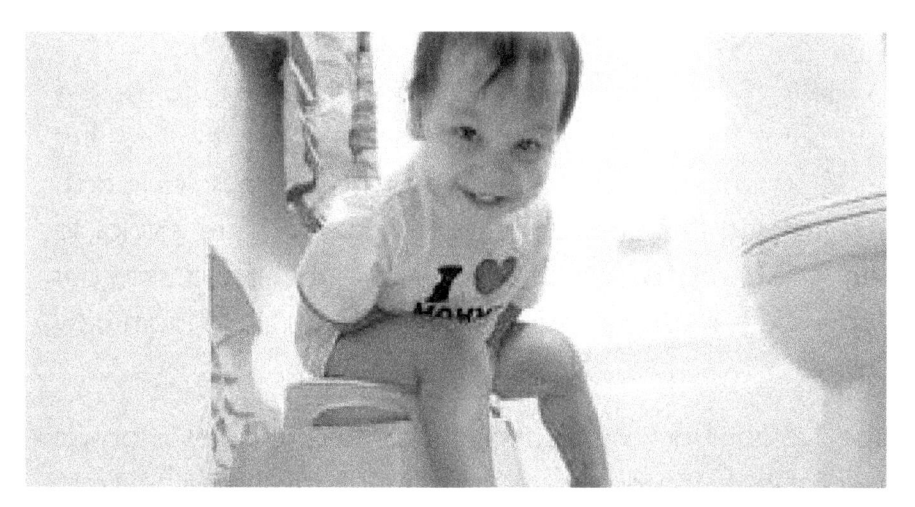

CHAPITRE 5

THE CHILD'S PREPARATION

Aside from recognizing the sensations of needing to use the restroom, getting there, and taking off one's clothes, the toddler must also learn to tense the sphincter muscles to gain control and then release them to excrete. There is a lot to learn. Gaining bowel and bladder control is a skill, but fortunately, most children love the opportunity to learn new things.

The typical learning progression for these abilities is bowel regularity or having bowel movements at the same time, followed by bowel control. Daytime bladder control normally follows though it may occur concurrently with bowel control in some toddlers. Last but not least is bladder control at night.

Begin teaching potty-training phrases.

When you decide it's time to start toilet training, there are a few things you can do to make the transition from diapers to underwear go more smoothly. Teach your youngster some potty-related terms, such as "pee," "poop," and "I need to go."

Before you start potty training, start reacting to your child's soiled diapers with words that emphasize how unpleasant it is to poop in a diaper. Make no mistake about it. Talk them through the process of going to the potty (pulling down trousers, sitting, pooping or peeing, pulling up pants, washing hands) several times. Make it commonplace.

Begin to make diaper-changing time-consuming.

When your child begins to express discomfort with a dirty diaper, try to make changing his diaper as inconvenient for him as it is for you, so that using the potty appears less demanding in comparison. Begin by showing your child what normal (unpadded) underwear looks like. If you use cloth diapers, this stage is less important because your child will recognize and become uncomfortable with the sensation of a wet or dirty diaper much sooner.

A child who is continuously kept in disposable diapers would never learn to stay dry since he will never feel wet. It will take some time for him to grasp and dislike the feeling of being wet once he quits wearing disposables and begins wearing underwear, and for him to learn to recognize those feelings before going to pee.

Introduce your toddler to the bathroom/toilet.

Begin taking your child into the bathroom with you two or three weeks before commencing the real three-day potty training, to make him feel comfortable in the bathroom. You may leave a nice potty-training book or a cool new toy in the bathroom for him to use while sitting on the potty seat. Stay in the bathroom with your kid, even if he spends a long time, and applaud him for even attempting to use the toilet chair.

Allow your child to observe and discuss what other people are doing when using the restroom. Discuss how they utilize toilet paper and how they use fresh paper for each wipe.

Allow your youngster to practice flushing the toilet. If you're

When you're finished using the toilet, have your child flush it for you, waving goodbye to the poop. Allow him to view pee and feces in the toilet.

Experiment with flushing it.

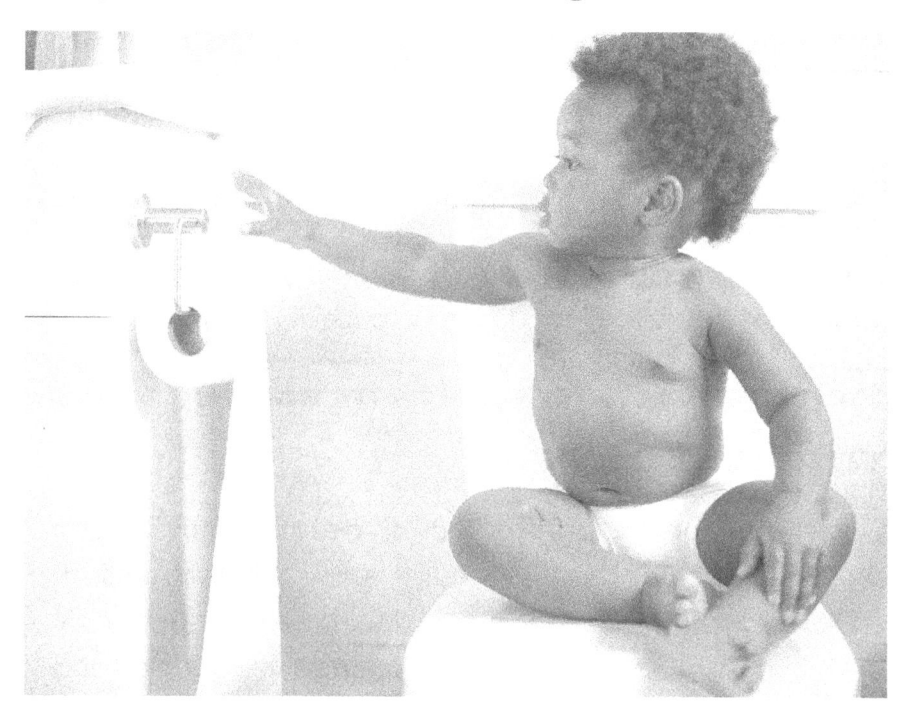

Bring out the potty chair.

Make the potty chair available to your kid early on so that he understands what it is for before you begin the three-day training. It will be much less difficult for your child if you have discussed the potty chair for a long time before the training and he is familiar with it, as opposed to introducing it to him just when you begin the training.

It's also a good idea to keep the potty chair in the bathroom rather than elsewhere in the house, such as in the child's bedroom or playroom, or the yard. Put the toilet chair in the bathroom that your toddler would normally use during the day if you live in a multi-story house.

It's a good idea to start demonstrating how to use the toilet chair by having your toddler sit on it before he's ready to use it. You can urge him to use the toilet seat with or without a diaper. Make sure his feet can reach the floor comfortably, or place something under his feet to help them reach.

Teach your youngster how to use the restroom in simple, everyday language. You could even empty his soiled diaper into the potty chair to explain its purpose.

Make your child's potty a relaxing and welcoming environment.

One week before the actual three-day potty-training process, make sure the toilet chair is in a well-lit restroom that your toddler can access. The toilet should be a friendly environment. Allow your toddler to examine, handle, and become acquainted with the potty chair. Tell him that this is his potty chair. Present it to him and discuss it with him, allowing him to try it out and become acquainted with it.

Encourage your youngster to use his or her potty chair whenever he or she needs to poop or pee. Tell him that he can let you know whenever he has to go to the restroom and that you will be available to take him there at any moment.

If your youngster is reluctant to use the toilet chair, don't force the subject. Maybe you had intended to start potty training but then something stressful happened.

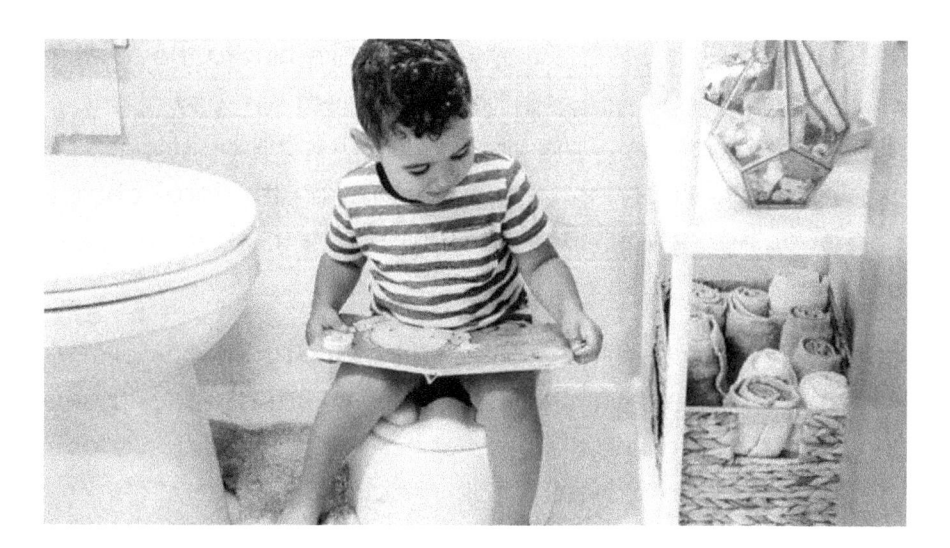

messing with your meticulously planned intentions If you try to potty train nevertheless, it will be tight and rushed, rather than casual and comfortable. If something comes up that disrupts your plans, reschedule the three-day block of time, and your youngster will resume interest once things are less stressful.

Make time for bathroom breaks.

Set your child on the potty chair when you think he needs to pee or defecate in the two weeks building up to the real three-day toilet training. You may have noticed a pattern, such as going roughly 30 minutes after eating or just after showering. However, these are only guidelines.

Don't take him to the potty if he shows no signs of needing to go.

Even if your toddler is still wearing diapers, you can show him where his bowel motions go before starting training.

Show him how to use the potty chair. Take him to the toilet chair whenever he poops in his diaper, seat him down, and dump the diaper into the potty chair. This will assist him in making the connection between sitting on the toilet chair and pooping, as well as understanding the purpose of the potty chair.

After you've emptied the potty chair into the bathroom toilet, you can allow your child to flush it to see where it goes (but don't force him to if he's terrified of the toilet). If the idea is for the toddler to associate bodily functions with the chair, having him sit on the potty chair fully clad is not as beneficial. It's customary for little boys to start off sitting on the toilet chair to pee, and then later learn to stand up once potty training is completed, usually when they wish to mimic their father or older brothers.

Setting your youngster on the potty chair when he doesn't need to go has been proved to be ineffective. It's best not to make your kid sit on the potty for extended periods because it will feel more like a punishment than a release.

Install a low step or stool near the bathroom sink so your toddler can wash his hands. Teach him how to wash his hands.

After using the restroom, wash your hands. Make it a habit to ask him if he has washed his hands and to lead him through the process with soap and water while you speak him through it. This might be an enjoyable hobby that your youngster incorporates into his daily routine.

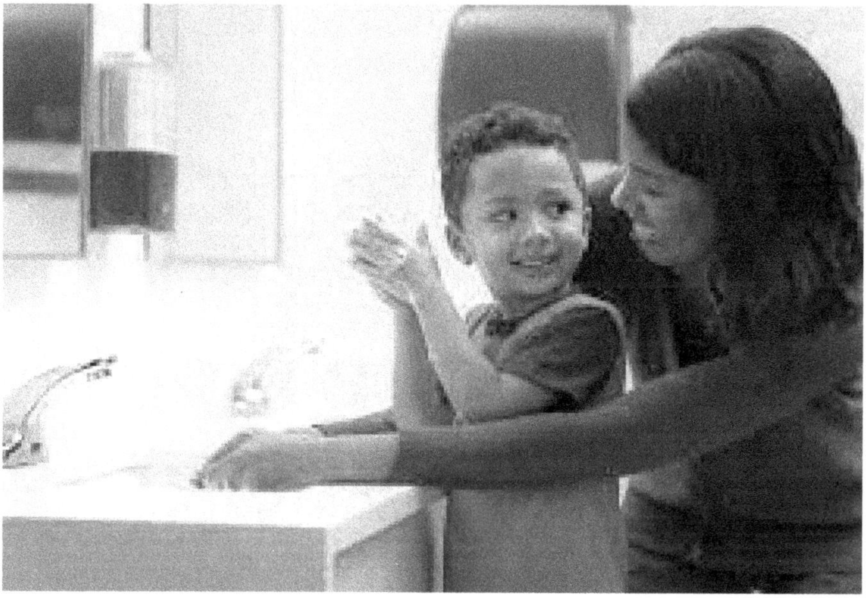

CHAPITRE 6

CALENDAR FOR POTTY-TRAINING

Set aside three consecutive days.

Make a note of them on your calendar. Keep in mind that the three days should not be sandwiched between major events or occasions that need a significant amount of labor and attention. Unless you have extra time off work, a three-day weekend like Labour Day or Memorial Day is usually the best time.

Don't plan on traveling anyplace throughout these three days. Allow yourself to concentrate on potty training because consistency is the key to success. Plan ahead of time how normal errands will be completed on certain days. Reschedule your child's childcare so that he is at home the entire time.

Make a list of activities that you and your toddler can do together.

During the three days of toilet training, you can schedule some activities outside, keeping in mind that you need to be able to hurry into the potty frequently, but it's preferable to largely plan on being inside.

inside. Spend most of your time in the house in an area with an easy-to-clean floor. Prepare by gathering books, colored pencils, markers, playdough, puzzles, toys, and television shows. You must keep your youngster occupied and pleasant during this three-day process, and three days inside with a toddler necessitates some ingenuity.

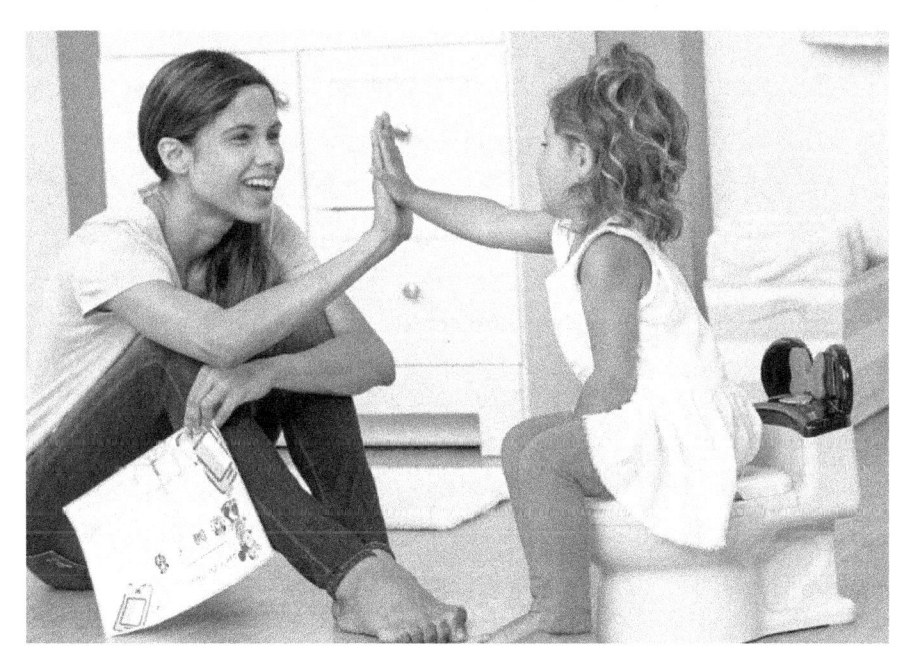

Do your laundry before you begin.

You should have clean linens, extra pajamas, and clothes on hand in case they have accidents once the training begins.

Increase the fiber content of your child's diet.

High-Fiber diets help prevent constipation by retaining adequate liquid in the stools, resulting in soft, easy-to-eliminate feces.

As a primary item in your child's daily meals, including a high-Fiber easy-to-eat grain. Most toddlers will happily consume Fiber-rich oat O's.

Serve yogurt with additional fiber for supper. Toddlers enjoy yogurt, and yogurts with added fiber are just as tasty and have the same smooth texture as regular yogurt.

Sandwiches should be made on high-Fiberwheat bread. Serve nut butter and jam on high-fiber wheat bread or whole-grain white bread to your child. White bread with whole grain contains less content than 100% whole wheat bread, but it contains more fiber than typical white bread.

An engaging element of your toddler's meals includes high-fiber veggies such as broccoli, sweet potatoes, spinach, and cabbage. Serve sweet potatoes with butter and brown sugar, or top a turkey sandwich with spinach or shredded cabbage.

Fiber-rich foods include beans, sweet potatoes, peas, tomatoes, and corn. Microwave a sweet potato for five to seven minutes. Peel it, then use a mold or cookie cutter to cut it into circles before serving. Steamed green beans or cauliflower should be served with ranch dressing for dipping. On a late spring day, chilled mashed peas are a refreshing delight.

Every day, give your child high-fiber fruits like apples, pears, and prunes. Natural goods are a simple way to incorporate fiber into your child's diet. When feasible, serve fruits and vegetables with the peel because the peel contains more fiber.

Prunes and apricots are high in fiber and have a laxative effect.

Serve grapes or cherry tomatoes cut in half with whole grain crackers. Slice an apple and put a thin layer of nut butter on top. Avocados are abundant in fiber and are a pleasant and sweet treat for children of all ages. Serve an array of cut-up fruits and vegetables on a brightly colored dish or even in an ice cube tray for variation.

Serve whole grain pasta and brown rice to your toddler instead of highly refined white pasta and rice.

Nutritionists suggest cutting back on cheese and other dairy products in \ our toddler's diet during the potty-training period since they can \shave a constipating effect. Also, offer your child a lot of water, which \ will help prevent constipation and will keep that bladder full, giving \ your little one lots of chances to practice!

A diet rich in high-fiber foods will not only make potty training easier \ for you and your toddler, but it's also a great way to present healthy \foods to your toddler and establish a pattern of eating healthily from \ an early age.

CHAPTER 7

EQUIPMENT ARSENAL

Have all the needed supplies ready before you begin the real three \ days of potty training.

High-Fiber food supplies and fluids

You should have more liquids on hand than your child typically drinks \in a day. Water is ideal. Besides water, an assortment of natural fruit \ and juices is also good.

Potty chair

Take your child with you to shop for the potty chair and let him pick out one he likes. It is best to start with a potty chair that sits on the \ floor and later if you want, you can move to one which sits on the \toilet seat of a normal toilet.

You can take the potty chair with you, even when you are out and \about. Kids become comfortable with their potty chairs and some \ prefer to use a public toilet when away from home. Try to figure out what works best for your toddler and go with it. In the end, your \toddler will figure out how to use both his potty chair and the toilet.

Take your child to the store with you, let him sit on various potty chairs if possible, and let him pick out the one he wants. As much as \she can, allow him to help you take it out of the store, put it in the car, \ and set it up in the bathroom when you get home.

Real underwear

You should have 10 to 20 pairs on hand. Take your child with you to \spick out some "big boy" underwear. Stay away from padded \underwear or pull-ups. As a part of working up enthusiasm in the \ spirit of your toddler, take him on a shopping trip a week before the \actual three-day training time, and let him pick out a couple of packs \ of underwear. A lot of times a toddler will get excited about using "big \boy" underwear with his favorite cartoon character on them.

The three-day strategy for potty training moves straight from diapers \ to regular clothes and underwear, with no pull-ups or training pants \ as a potty-training aid, since wearing pull-ups encourages \skids to pee in them. Disposable training pants are advertised as a \gentle introduction to normal underwear, but they aren't \effective.

Training pants may seem to be helpful at first since they keep you \ from having to deal with a mess on your floors, couches, and other \furniture, but they confuse toddlers and make them think it is \ okay to use them like diapers. For that reason, using training pants \ and softening works against potty-training progress.

Pull-ups are another item that delays potty-training progress.

They have for some time been criticized because they keep the child \ from feeling wet from accidents, thus slowing down the learning \ process. Sadly, they are regularly advertised for use as underwear \ for three and four-year-olds who are not yet potty trained, which \ further puts off developing the skills of controlling bodily functions.

Easy-wear clothing

Make sure your child's wardrobe is suitable for potty training. Try to \avoid overalls or clothes with buttons and snaps. Simple clothes that \ allow the child to easily undress himself are essential at this stage of \spotty training.

Moist baby wipes

You can keep wet wipes in the bathroom a few days ahead of \time so your toddler knows that they are for him to use. Wet wipes \offer a cleaner and more delicate wipe than toilet paper, but most \ baby wipes and other wet wipes are not made of biodegradable \ materials and can't be flushed down the toilet because they don't \disintegrate. There are some flushable wet wipes available, but \ some of them contain household cleaning agents that can be \aggravating if they contact the eyes.

There are also economical ways to make your wet wipes. A lot \ of mothers have learned how to make two rolls of wet wipes out of \ one roll of paper towels by cutting it in half and soaking the halves in \ a mixture of water, baby soap, and baby oil or almond oil. Then the \swipes are stored in an air and water-proof container and remain \moist for a month or two. When you look at the cost, it makes a lot of \ sense, and you can customize the scent.

Others make their homemade reusable baby wipes out of cloth.

Though that may sound gross to those who are used to using \disposable wipes, it saves money and is much better for \ the environment. Making reusable baby wipes from the best \available material will cost less than $60 for a set of 24 clothes that \ will last you from birth to potty training. Traditional wipes tend to cost \ about $4 for a pack of 80, which might last only seven days, running \sup a total cost of $208 every year!

When you make your baby wipes, you know exactly what is in \ the soap solution, so you know exactly what is touching your child's \ skin. Instead of the alcohol, fragrance, and chorine normally found in traditional baby wipes, custom-made wipes can be made with \entirely safe substances and paper towels. Homemade wipes are \durable and are the least aggravating to your toddler's skin.

Snacks, treats, and rewards

Come up with a reward system that matches your parenting style \ and doesn't conflict with what your toddler is used to from you. For \ instance, you might buy a gift bag with your toddler's favorite cartoon \character and fill it with "pee prizes" or "poop prizes." Coloring books, \ small toys, and individual Hershey's Kisses are examples of some of the \ these things. Or you could let your toddler pick a prize when he goes \poop and uses stickers and fruit snacks when he goes pee.

For some parents, Mini M&Ms are a big help in potty training. The \idea could be, that each time your child goes potty, he gets a few, but if \she wipes himself (which is a tremendous accomplishment), he is \rewarded with four or five. This helps a toddler to overcome the \ difficulty of not wanting to poop on the potty because learning how to \swipe himself is yucky.

If your child reacts well to stickers or stars on a chart, you could use \ that method too. A reward chart can be a useful tool to use so the \toddler can see a visual indication of how well he is progressing.

Some parents reward their child with a new book, toy, or other gifts \ when he has stayed dry or used the potty for a certain amount of \time.

For others, trips to the park or an extra bedtime story are effective \rewards. Figure out what works best for your child. Reinforce your \child's efforts with verbal praise, for example, "You're doing great!

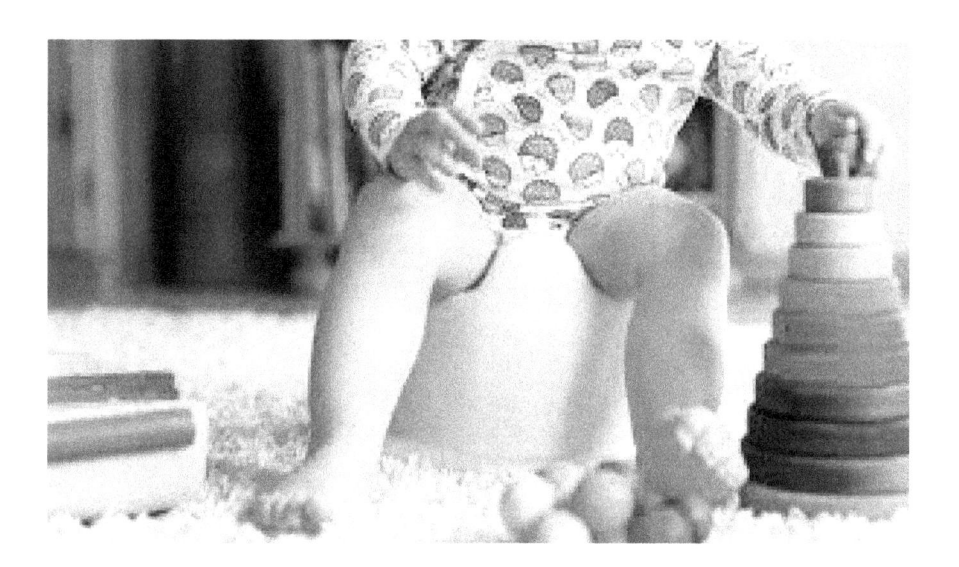

You're learning how to use the potty just like big kids do!" Even if \your toddler doesn't do everything successfully, give praise for any \ part of the procedure that he can do.

Cleaning supplies \You will also need to have supplies on hand for cleaning up \accidents; for example, cleaning rags, soap or disinfectant, and a \plastic bucket.

CHAPTER 8

THREE-DAY POTTY-TRAINING METHOD

The rule that makes the Three-Day Method effective

Each child is different. Even among siblings, each child will show \different signs of readiness, react differently to training, and learn in \his or her particular way, which then should be encouraged. But \ just because things don't seem to be working at first the way we \ expected, that doesn't mean that "the technique doesn't work" and \ that you should throw out the whole strategy.

This is one reason to read through this book a few times BEFORE \ starting the Three-Day technique, and not while you're in the middle \ of it. After you give it a while to stew in your mind as you watch your

toddler's reactions and disposition, by the time you start the three- \day training you will know the concepts "by heart" and won't simply have to go "by the book."

Once you read through this material a few times, you'll know how to \personalize the ideas in the three-day technique. You will be able to \know in what areas to be flexible and in what areas to be firm and \consistent. For example, you may change ideas about what kind of \prizes to use and how, but will know that you must be firm about \using normal clothes and not pull-ups after you get rid of the diapers.

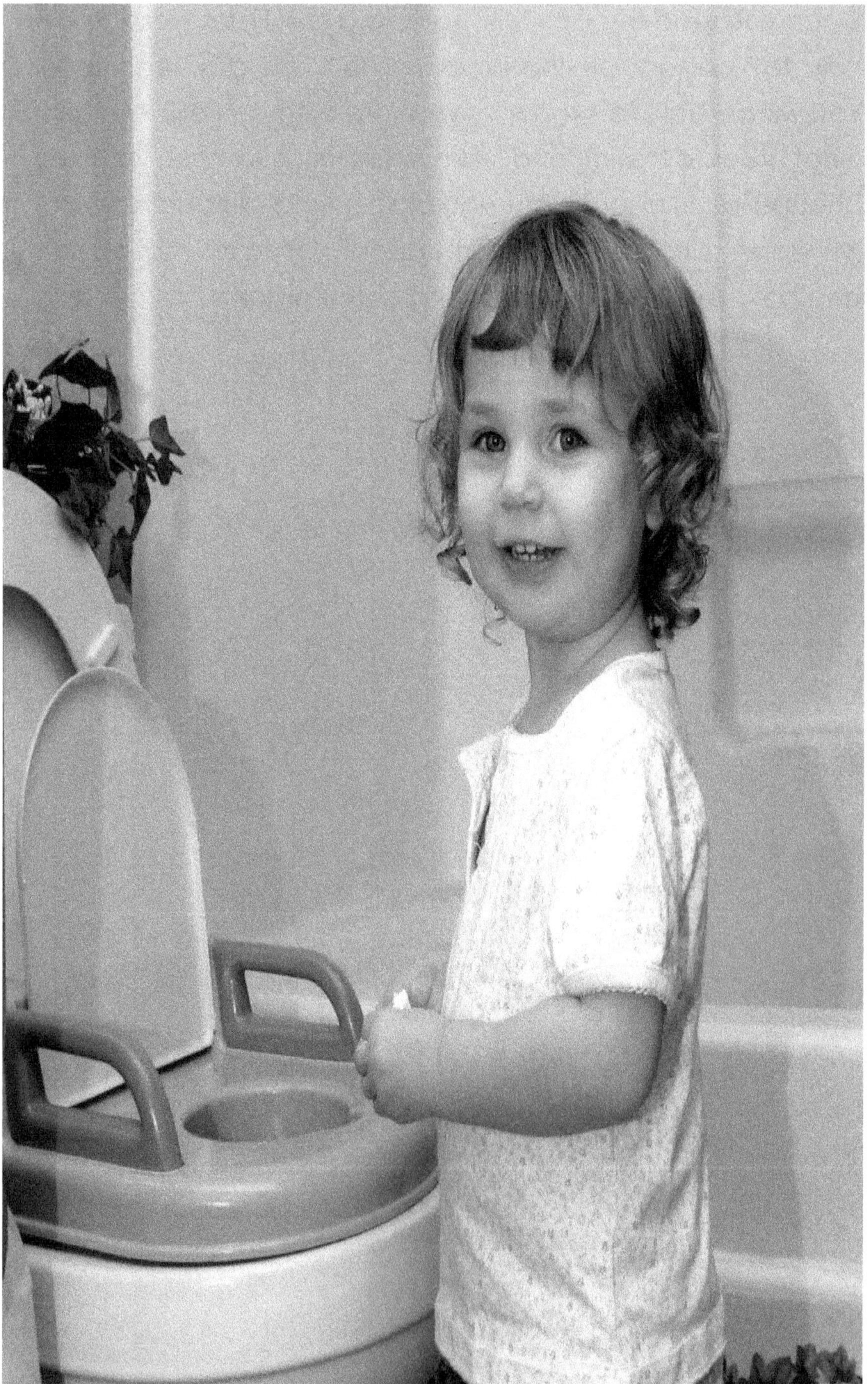

At the very center of what is firm and what is flexible, \certain principles make the three-day potty-training technique \effective. They apply to every child, without much variation because \ of the kid's personality. Be prepared to never fall short in the areas \ of:

Persistence

Consistency

Patience

Positivity

Love

No discipline, punishment, or negative correction \ strategies

Accidents are going to happen, so be ready for them. Even children \ who have used the potty effectively for a long time sometimes have \accidents. Try not to make your child feel bad for having an accident.

Scolding your child will make the potty-training process take longer, not less time. Keep this in mind when you feel frustrated.

Instead of criticizing your toddler, tell him to let you know when he \needs to go pee so you can take him to the potty straight away. Remember that encouragement is the most effective strategy, so continue to praise your toddler for a job well done or for attempting.

When a youngster refuses to use the potty, he or she will defecate or pee instantly if the diaper is removed. Don't be disheartened. Even though it may be tempting to revert to diapers or pull-ups, continue to use regular clothing, even during nighttime training. It will all be worthwhile in the end.

Getting your toddler ready ahead of time will surely assist, which is why it is a good idea to help your toddler become familiar with the potty for two weeks before beginning the real training. Even if you are a parent or caregiver with physical restrictions that prevent you from participating in some areas of potty training, you can still participate.

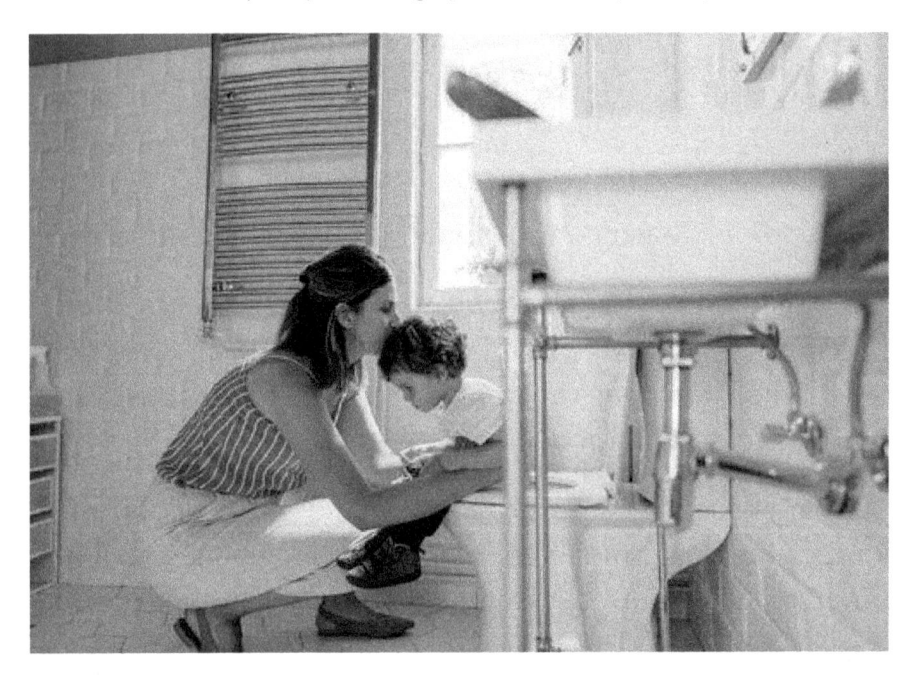

Be involved in the teaching, rewarding, and other non-physical aspects of the process.

The First Day

The first day may be the most difficult, particularly for working women who are unfamiliar with remaining at home with their children. It's not easy for stay-at-home moms either, but in either scenario, the benefits will far surpass the effort for any parent who is prepared. But it takes a lot of perseverance and patience.

You should constantly monitor your youngster for signs that they need to use the restroom. You may first miss the indications until they begin to fade. If this is the case, as soon as you notice your child starting to go, rush him to the potty so he may finish the process there. As he walks, talk to him about how he feels the need to go.

"Did you feel like you needed to pee?" When you feel like that, it's time to use the restroom." Be calm and soothing.

Give your youngster a treat every time he uses the toilet, no matter how infrequently.

The toilet should be located in the bathroom.

In the long run, your child should associate the potty chair with the need to pee or poop in the toilet rather than in another location such as the yard or in front of the TV. When your child is seated on the potty, make sure his feet are comfortable on the floor or a stool. Review the terminology you chose previously to help your child understand how to talk about restroom fundamentals.

Breakfast should be eaten by both you and your child.

Plenty of high-fiber foods, cereals, fruits, and drinks. Juice is preferable to dairy, which just results in harder stools.

Set the tone for the day's training.

When you take your child's diaper off when he wakes up, talk to him about how that is the final diaper he will wear while you clean him up and get him ready for the day. Dress him in simple clothes.

Instead of full-body jumpsuits, choose loose-fitting pants with a flexible belt.

In a warm area, you may only want to clothe your child in a shirt and underpants to get him on the potty faster and avoid accidents. Some parents prefer the "bare bottom" method, although it is better for the child to become used to wearing clothes while still desiring to use the potty.

Naptime

It is beneficial to take your child potty before and after he sleeps. There may be some accidents at first, but he will soon figure out how to keep dry during naptime and how to wake you up when he needs to go at night, or he may even surprise you by going by himself.

Your child's ability to keep dry during naps and at night will improve as he becomes more accustomed to using the bathroom during the day.

Night-time training may occur sooner than expected, but don't be concerned if it does not. Even if your child is regularly clean and dry during the day, it may take him a few weeks to learn evening training. Boys, in particular, often take their time developing the physical capacity to contain their pee while sleeping.

The second day

Continue to follow the same recommendations from Day One, using the insights obtained through observing your child's actions and reactions.

On Day Two, you can go outside for an hour after your child has peed in the potty.

Try not to get frustrated by accidents or if your youngster does not seem to understand. A youngster who is used to using disposable diapers may put you to the test to see if they can return to wearing diapers that are less demanding for them. Try not to back down; instead, stay positive and pleasant, and they will soon realize that you are not going to give in.

It's Day Two, but don't push your child. Relax and allow him to learn at his rate; he's getting the hang of it now.

He was there yesterday. Keep him engaged by talking to him and telling him stories, but the most important thing your child needs at this stage is to know that you approve of him, so continue to praise him for his efforts and tell him what a good job he's doing.

It's not uncommon for Day Two to feel exactly like Day One, but it's also possible that your child will begin to get into the swing of things and have a few accidents. There may still be some near misses, but hopefully not as many total disasters. On Day Two, your toddler may learn how to recognize the need to go potty so that he can go on time.

Your child may be surprised at first that he knows what to do, but he may still feel uncomfortable and try to hold his excrement instead of going. However, if you see any of these symptoms, place your child on the potty and give him a book to read to help him relax, and he should be able to go easily. Then you might say to him, "That's fantastic! You've got it now!" Once a child can successfully poop in the potty, the rest should be easier, but be consistent and stick to the training plan.

The third day

On Day Three, you can go outside for an hour in the morning and another hour in the afternoon, just after your child pees. This reinforces to him that he needs to pee before going outside, and it allows him ample time to come back into the house and be near the potty before he goes again.

When going outside, your toddler should simply wear a shirt, underpants, and loose-fitting pants. Even when outside, avoid using diapers or pull-ups since they provide a signal to the child's brain that there is anything there to capture the feces or urine, which can lead to regressions.

On Day Three, you may be in for a surprise, especially if you began the Three-Day Method without a lot of pressure from high expectations. Instead of Day Three being the same as Days One and Two, your child may suddenly grasp it and have no accidents all day!

But don't give up if your youngster still doesn't seem to be getting it at this time. His brain, body, and muscles are all catching on. Simply maintain your confidence while assisting your youngster in remembering the elements of the training that he can perform. Continue to engage in things that you both like in between trips to the restroom, such as reading books, playing games, eating ice cream, baking, and eating cookies.

As the potty becomes more appealing to your youngster, his or her resistance will weaken. He may begin to utilize verbal cues such as "Mommy, potty" rather than only signals, and he may joyfully sit on the potty. Even if nothing occurs, he is at least sitting there and trying. It also helps if an older brother comes home from school and encourages him.

Day Three could also be a disaster, and it may appear that all progress made on Days One and Two has been lost. But don't give up hope. At the end of the day, ask your husband or another adult to watch your child while you step outside to vent and, if necessary, cry. This will enable you to refocus on how to apply incentives more effectively.

CHAPITRE 9

WHEN NOTHING ELSE WORKS

(A step-by-step procedure based on a true story)

Nothing seems to work at times. All methods and customary advice appear to fail. It occurs, and you are not alone. There is no single plan that works 100% of the time, but your love as a parent is the key that unlocks the door to success. Keep it in mind.

Let me tell you about my kid, Bobby. His tale is our story, and perhaps someone will find it useful because of the parallels to their situation. And perhaps our experience will assist you in overcoming one of the most challenging difficulties for parents and children: potty training.

Bobby was born 35 weeks early. He had to be resuscitated, and the doctors were able to save his life. However, due to all of the antibiotics he had to take, he developed bowel movement issues. He had a lot of constipation difficulties when he was two years old, and he remembered it for a long time.

These memories of constipation posed a dilemma when we began potty training. Bobby rapidly learned to urinate in the potty without any assistance.

But he was terrified of sitting down and pooping on the potty.

We begged, pleaded, promised, and provided rewards... but nothing worked: fear, tension, tears, and even enemas.

Bobby was already out of diapers, but he was terrified of pooping on the potty. As a result, he would keep it for a few days. Even when he tried to poop, he failed.

Our fight lasted for several months. I almost gave up hope at times, fearing that our son might suffer from severe psychological trauma. But, thanks to his previous experience and support, my spouse was there for me and didn't let me down.

As a result, we studied hundreds of books and tried every well-known tip and remedy. Finally, after two months of hard work, our efforts were rewarded. Bobby peed on the toilet by himself!

And now he goes to the potty with great delight. You should see his proud expression! :)

So, what did we do to assist him? There wasn't simply one straightforward remedy, but rather a combination of seven crucial ideas.

They are as follows:

No-stress.

Don't worry about placing too much pressure on your youngster. Try not to panic and try to let the matter go.

The proper equipment.

We switched out the potty chair, attempting to find the most comfortable shape.

In my opinion, it is advisable to purchase a potty chair that does not have any toys or musical devices. You don't want your child to think of the potty as a toy since he can start playing with it and become sidetracked from the potty-training process.

As previously stated, you can try selecting and purchasing a potty chair with your child. Allow him to choose which one he wants to utilize.

We then placed the potty in a location that our boy felt comfortable with. You might even need to keep the toilet chair in your living room for a while! If your youngster feels at ease there, go with it! Believe me, it's worthwhile!

I'm drinking a lot of water.

Please keep one of the most crucial aspects of healthy body growth in mind: drinking. And it is critical that your child not only consume juice and milk, but also water!!!

It's critical to offer your child a drink of water and then put him on the potty as he wakes up, especially in the morning.

If your youngster isn't used to drinking water, start with little steps.

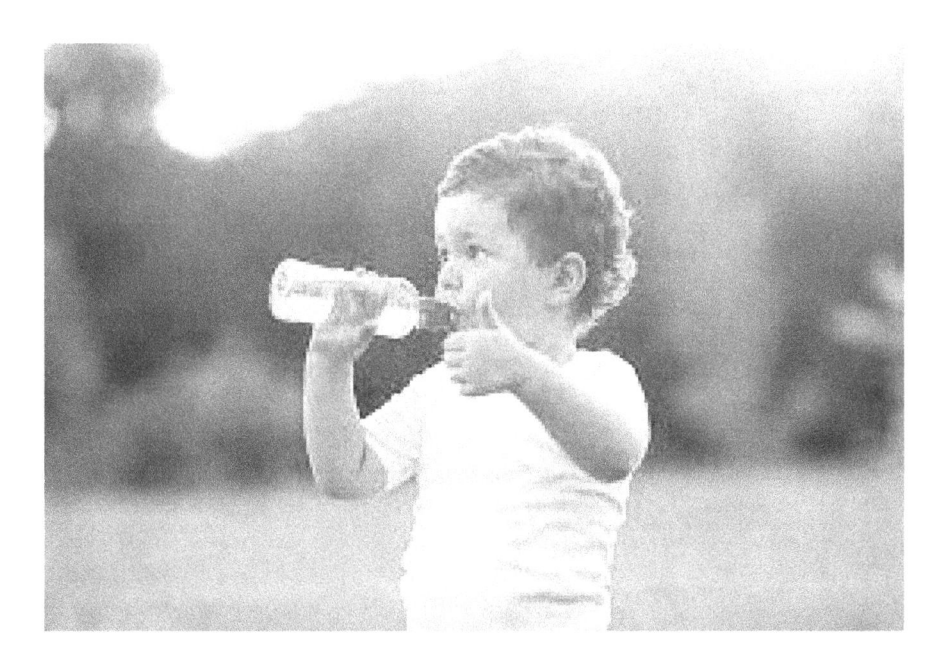

Explain how important this is and how it will help him be as strong, courageous, and swift as his favorite cartoon character. You might even turn it into a game.

Depending on his weight, your toddler should drink two to three cups of water every day. You could get him his convenient water bottle, which he could choose himself.

Routine.

It's easy to become preoccupied with getting your toddler to poop in the morning.

After all, getting into a pattern will make the procedure of going poop at preschool or daycare easier in the future.

But that isn't the most crucial consideration. Bobby, for example, preferred to poop in the evenings at first.

He used to always wait until after dark. He eventually became more comfortable with the potty and now uses it anytime he wants.

Every time your youngster goes to use the potty he should sense your \ support. Don't push him and allow him as much time as he requires, but don't let him sit for too long without results.

Foods are high in fiber.

Pay close attention to nutrition, as we did. Our son adored bread, muffins, chocolate, and cakes, all of which caused constipation and exacerbated his potty issues.

That's why I compiled a list of meals that would be beneficial to my child's health and stimulate his digestive system.

We started giving our son more veggies and fruit by replacing white flour with rye flour and wheat flour cookies with oats. Allow your youngster to consume even two spoonfuls of vegetables, and they will be quite beneficial and will do their tasks. Here's an example of my menu.

Here are some of the foods that were beneficial to us: Beets, carrots, cauliflower, and broccoli are all examples of root vegetables. Apples, plums, and watermelons are all in season. Lean fish and meat, baked potatoes, porridges, cereals, cereal flakes, dried fruit, salad dressing with olive oil Kefir/buttermilk, yogurt, and low-fat cottage cheese are all good options.

The doctor advised us to take baby probiotics and vitamin courses.

In our instance, they appeared to be a suitable option and to be of assistance.

YouTube video examples

It was fascinating to witness how my spouse assisted our son with his potty training. He showed him many videos.

My buddy suggested that I show our son a video of children using the potty. She claimed she did it to help her young daughter learn to use the toilet. But such videos did not appeal to our youngsters in the least.

So, Daddy chose some "special" videos for him. Knowing how much he adores animals such as tigers, cheetahs, and other predators, my husband found and showed him footage of these animals pooping on YouTube.

Our son was quite intrigued, and my husband explained that pooping isn't frightening, that it's simple, and that it doesn't hurt. The following time our kid sat on the potty, and he begged to watch the video again.

Bobby was fascinated by the excrement of these creatures. It was amusing, but it also made us pleased. Bobby soon began to try to go himself.

Rewards.

Our final tactical and strategic step was to reward our son's efforts. He rewarded himself after each successful toilet trip.

I immediately received a gift. We gave him toys, candy, and cookies as a reward.

It's critical to be reasonable here. You can give a tiny incentive, such as one or two biscuits or a small toy. Just enough to make the child pleased and motivate him further.

Poop and hug together.

Bobby struggled at first to push and poop. He was continually concerned about his ability to complete the task. We devised a simple solution to assist him to overcome his worry and fear.

Remember how powerful a parent's love was?

It was instinctual and came from the bottom of my heart. But it was quite beneficial.

What exactly did we do? When our son was on the toilet, we simply sat next to him and cuddled him. Just a few hugs let him sense our support, get rid of his nervousness, and push as hard as he needed to.

He then discovered that he could simply use the restroom. He learned the essential abilities and reflexes and began to accomplish things on his own.

But those hugs were crucial for him in the beginning.

Of course, the embraces do not have to come from everyone in the family. It might be just you, your husband, or someone your son trusts.

Ritual Farewell.

During potty training, our family established a humorous routine. Our youngsters needed to perceive the process as a game. He became so engrossed in it that he forgot about his concerns and mental distress.

So, as our son performed "his business," we deposited the poop in the potty and shouted, "Bye-bye, poop!" Say hello to your buddies for us!" and our youngster hit the button, flushing it into the toilet. It was entertaining to watch him enjoy the entire procedure.

Repeat.

You'll feel like you're in seventh heaven the first time everything goes right, but it's critical to build on your success. Repeat the process for a few weeks.

Your efforts will undoubtedly bear fruit! One day, your child will amaze you by doing everything without your assistance.

Patience.

You may experience hopelessness at times. You'll be angry with your child and with yourself at times. But don't give in to despair.

Don't express your disappointment or be upset with your youngster.

Your child is aware of your disappointment and anger, and he is as concerned as you are.

If you need to cry, cry; if you need to yell, scream. But do it in another room where your youngster cannot see or hear you. He needs your help, understanding, and love.

So, this process may take you a few days or a few weeks. Be patient and follow your heart. Use all of the advice I've given you, and you will undoubtedly succeed in this vital family challenge.

WATER IS THE KEY IN CHAPTER 10

Your child's body will require more water as he grows and begins eating solid foods. Additionally, fluid loss increases due to the child's increased activity.

Water aids in digestion. It prevents constipation and facilitates bowel movements. That is precisely what we require for potty training!

Every day, a child requires three to five cups of water. Water that is not carbonated. Juices, soda, milk, milkshakes, smoothies, tea, and other beverages

Chocolate milk and other similar beverages are not permitted.

How does one go about teaching a child to drink water?

1. Children mimic their parents' actions. Drink plenty of water, and your youngster will want to do the same.

2. Rituals are appealing to children. Begin a "water" routine by drinking a glass of water as soon as you get up and again a few hours before night.

Always have your youngster drink water after he or she has pooped!

3. Make water available at all times. Always provide your child with water everywhere he goes. Keep water bottles throughout the house, particularly in the bedroom and living room.

Children are so preoccupied with playing that they sometimes forget about thirst. If your toddler dislikes the taste of water, add some lemon or lime slices to improve the flavor.

4. Tell your youngster as often as possible about the importance of water to his body. It is not only the source of health but also of beauty.

5. A glass of water before and after going for a walk.

6. Allow your youngster to drink water from a lovely bottle that features a beloved cartoon character or a brightly colored bottle.

7. Always provide your youngster with water anytime you serve him sweets, chocolate, cookies, or desserts. Drinking water after eating sweets will help keep his teeth clean, and we all want our children's teeth to be clean and healthy.

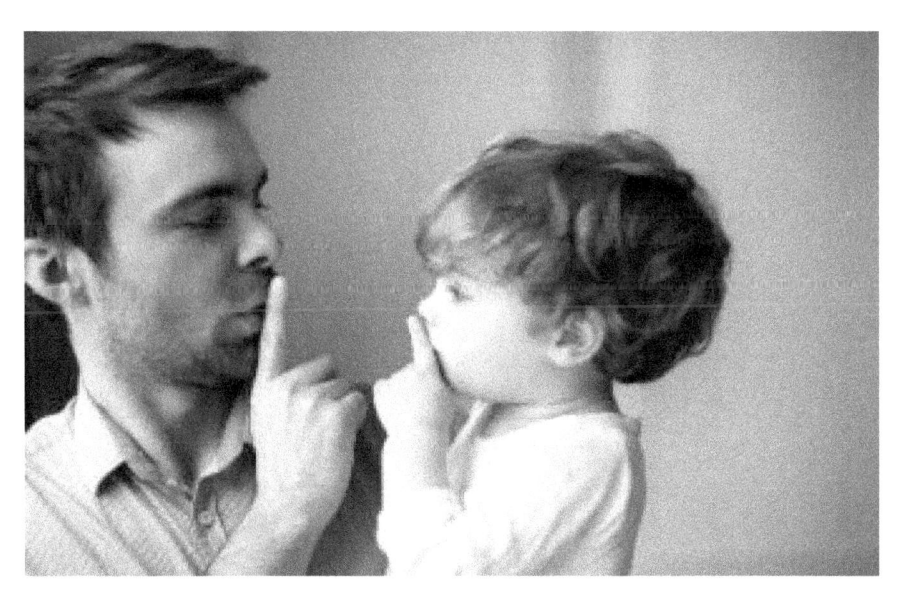

CHAPTER 11

SPECIALITIES OF BOY POTTY TRAINING

When you believe your child is ready, concentrate on the time. Make sure your child's routine is well established. If he has just begun daycare or has a younger brother or sister, he may be less sensitive to change or be too eager to take on this new challenge.

Allow him to observe and learn.

Little ones learn through imitation. Going to the toilet is thus a natural initial step for adults. And here is where having a male at home comes in handy. Following his father, uncle, or a family friend to the toilet to see him pee can help your boy become more familiar with the idea. He might notice that Dad and Mom do not use

In the same way, the toilet will provide you with the opportunity to explain how tiny boys pee.

Purchase the proper equipment.

Most experts advise you to get a pottychair that your toddler can make her own and that will reaure him more than using a huge toilet (many youngsters are afraid to fall inthe toilet, and this anxiety can slow down

If you wish to buy a child's toilet seat that fits on your toilet seat, ensure that it is comfortable and securely fastened. If you choose this option, you will also need to purchase a step stool so that your child can easily climb up and down to and from the toilet when he has to use it and can stabilize his legs while seated. Another wonderful way to facilitate learning is to find a nice book or video that explains how to use the toilet.

Assist your child in becoming acquainted with the toilet.

At this point, your boy should be comfortable using the toilet. Begin by helping him understand that the potty chair or the potty eater belongs to him. You may personalize it by writing his name on it or letting him decorate it with stickers.

A week later, you can suggest that he remove his pants and underwear or diaper. Don't force him if he resists. This will simply create a power struggle that could derail the entire operation. If your child has a favorite doll or toy, use it to teach him how to use the restroom. Children enjoy seeing their favorite toy come to life, and the experience will have a greater impact than if it came from you. Some parents even create a miniature potty for the doll in this way, everyone has their potty!

Buy him a big boy's underwear.

Draw your son's attention to the benefits of being clean by taking him on a special shopping excursion to buy his first pair of real underpants! Tell him he can choose the ones he wants (briefs or boxers with beloved cartoons or superheroes are always popular).

Talk about this shopping day in advance so he is interested in the idea of becoming large enough to go Potty and wear real" clothes.

underwear, just like his father or older siblings.

Create a learning schedule for toilet training.

Your ability to leave your child without a diaper will be determined by your daily schedule. If you need someone else to monitor your child while you are at work, you must communicate your strategy to the daycare staff or babysitter. You will need to choose between Diapers and underwear. If not using diapers is a practical option, many professionals and parents choose to put children directly into washable underwear, which allows the youngster to feel wet right away.

Of course, this will necessitate cleaning up in the event of an accident.

If you can't settle on a method, consult with your pediatrician. It will be necessary to use disposable diapers or training pants at night and on lengthy travels for some time.

Educate him to pee sitting down first, then standing up. Because pooping and peeing frequently occur at the same time, it makes more sense to teach your child to sit down first so he understands that everything goes into the toilet. In this manner, he will not try to play with his pee and learn to aim, while he is supposed to focus just on measuring the basics of using the potty.

When your son is comfortable on his potty or eating, have him try the standing position on his little stool so it is at the proper height level. There is no reason to rush items. He can stay as long as he wants. If he appears hesitant to stand up, float a small amount of toilet paper or another small object in the toilet bowl as a target. Expect to clean the toilet!

Leave your boy half-dressed.

Your child can learn when he needs to go to the toilet by remaining only partially dressed. Place the Potty somewhere accessible from where he plays, and encourage him to use it on occasion.

Watch for signals (if he puts his hand on his privates, squirms, or bounces around), then suggest that he use the restroom. You can do this over several consecutive days, in the evening when the family is all together, or just on the weekend, as you see fit. The longer your child spends without being fully clothed, the faster he will learn.

CHAPITRE 12

REWARDS AND CELEBRATION

TO ACHIEVE SUCCESS

It is critical to understand the distinction between a reward and a bribe. The line can become a little blurry here, but the essential difference is this: A reward comes after the conduct you're attempting to reinforce, whereas a bribe comes before it. Also, a reward should be delivered as soon as feasible after the behavior that is being rewarded, to establish a strong association between the behavior and the positive reinforcement.

Do you know how excited you get when your child or daughter says they're ready to start potty training? The signal you've been patiently waiting for? Maybe not forever, but for a long time. Some children, especially those under the age of three, can be encouraged to use the restroom if a reward is offered afterward. Stickers, if your child I ready to potty train anyway small Prize a trip to the Library or the Park or the playing a beloved game together may work well the reward motivates a child to continue practicing abilities that would otherwise be uninteresting to him.

Every child will be simpler to inspire with rewards and will more gladly complete the work at hand for a small Potty-training Celebration after he's done. Here are some Potty-Training Celebration Ideas if prizes or fun motivation work for your child. Potty training is a significant thing for both you and your child, and using a reward system is an excellent approach to encourage potty-training success.

1. A chart with stickers

A young child finds it quite exciting to select a ticker and place it in a specific location. And watching the stickers collect over time is a nice visual reminder of what a fantastic job they're doing!

2. Potty treat jar

Fill a jar with your favorite little candy. Whether it's quicker jellybeans, M&M's, or skittle, you may discover that a small amount of candy can go a long way toward encouraging your youngster to stay dry during the day.

3. Potty rewards

If candy isn't your thing, go to the dollar shop and make a potty prize box. Every time your child pees or poops in the toilet, he gets to choose a new toy to play with.

Alternatively, offer larger items as an incentive for earning stickers on your child's sticker chart. If kids use the potty all week, they might get to pick out a toy at the store during the weekend.

If your child enjoys having friends around, you could allow him to have a playdate on Saturday if he stays dry all day on Friday. Let him choose what the family eats for supper if he only has one accident during the day. You know your child better than anyone, and you know what will motivate him to use the restroom.

Parental Guidance: Begin small!

When deciding what reward to offer for potty training, parents that have gone before you will advise you to start modest. If your child enjoys the "reward" of flushing the toilet every time he uses it, there is no need to waste your money on toys or candy.

If your one is so excited that he just wants one piece of candy when he pees, there's no need to give him ten. Start small and gradually increase your reward if necessary to motivate your children. This will save you from having to go to the toy store every time your child poos on the potty!

CHAPITRE 13

REPEAT EAT, PLAY, POOP

Potty training a child successfully and rapidly does not happen by chance. Rather, parents who want to potty train a child in a matter of days must arm themselves with a time-tested system and a well-thought-out plan of action that builds their self-confidence and allows them to tap into their strength while avoiding the most common and costly pitfall.

It is important to go over all of the potty-training tips for boys, but if you have a strong-willed child and are convinced that potty training him will become a test of will, or if you are already frustrated after one or more unsuccessful attempts at potty training your child, know that you are not alone.

As a parent, you should be aware that there is no set time for toilet training for boys. To look for preparedness to use the potty, you should study your child's general inclinations. The process may be exhausting, but patience is required. Tell and demonstrate to your son how to use the toilet. You may use a doll to demonstrate different potty habits.

Your child will need you to be confident, calm, and focused on him during the scheduled potty training. Decide when you want to start training and free your calendar for a few days within that time. Make sure there are no too stressful events in your child's life during potty training time. If your family life is currently difficult or chaotic, stop training your little potty trainee until things calm down.

It is critical to repeat the potty-training procedure until your child is toilet-trained.

Prepare your child. Discuss with him what you intend to educate him about.

Allow your child to observe you using the restroom. Modeling is crucial!

Give your child plenty of fluids during the day of potty training.

Take him to the toilet chair every one to two hours.

Something will happen on the potty chair at some point!

Make a huge deal out of his success. Be matter-of-fact about everything else.

Repeat this method until your child has received toilet training.

Realize that while initial training may only take a few days, making the process a habit will take months.

If your child has a lot of accidences, it is often effective to let him wear underwear but then put a pull-up on top of the underwear. Even if he has an accident his underpants will become Wet, which he will feel.

Pull-ups frequently absorb so much that the child does not feel the sensation of being wet, which is an important part of potty training. The reason you put a pull-up over his underwear is to keep his clothes, and his classroom, if he is in school, from getting wet Teacher, will appreciate it!

Remind the teachers to encourage your child to use the restroom regularly. Children become so engrossed in their play that they frequently forget to go to the bathroom.

the bathroom until too late Teacher should encourage the child to at least try to go and should praise them for doing so.

It is preferable in the classroom if youngsters are allowed to use the restroom whenever they need to. Some children go to the toilet repeatedly while potty training, which is fine. Over time, the child will gain a better understanding when he repeats this process when he truly needs to go, and the frequency will decrease.

CHAPITRE 14

MANAGING ACCIDENTS

Accidents must be handled quietly and gently. You must also learn to read your boy's signs to know when he needs to use the restroom. It will take both of you working together to make potty training successful.

Let's pretend everything is going swimmingly. Your little one appears to have mastered potty training, and you believe you've said goodbye to diapers for good. But then he starts having accidents again, and you wonder what went wrong. Accidents occur frequently because a child is having too much fun playing or doing an activity and just does not want to stop to hurry to the bathroom.

Rest assured that many children experience potty training regression - it is quite normal. However, you should consider if your child was ever truly potty trained in the first place. It is fairly frequent for an occasional setback in the first day, month, or even years of potty training However, a youngster who has multiple accidents every day and does not appear to care about them should not be considered "potty trained." Consider whether your child is ready to potty train. Start looking for a way to get back on track if he wants to. If

Notify your pediatrician when he or she believes your child is ready.

If your child has an accident, don't be upset; doing so can make your little one more anxious, which can lead to further potty problems. Do everything you can to be positive, even if it means going back to having children and possibly having to use diapers due to toilet-training issues.

When you check to see if your child is dry, applaud and cheer if he is. If he isn't, then remain nonjudgmental and remark, " "ops. You were involved in an accident. Let's use the restroom." Remember to stay positive and never yell or reprimand your child. You want your children to feel empowered and not fear being punished if they make a mistake.

You won't be able to halt the setbacks unless you address the underlying issue. Try to discover the causes of the regression, since addressing them would assist the child in returning to where he was. For example, many children begin having accident during times of transition that may cause tre, such as starting a new school or welcoming a new sibling. If that is the case, chances are your child will need potty training again once her lives settle down. Even if your child gets through the day without incident, he may still have nightmares at night. Many children are not dry at night for years after being dry during the day. Accident potty-training can also be caused by medical concerns, with constipation being a common one. If a youngster has trouble making a bowel movement, he may teer clear of the potty entirely to avoid having to pooh and strain. Make sure your child is getting enough fiber and water, but if he is afraid of pooping on the toilet, play games or read stories with him while he sits on the toilet to make it more pleasurable.

Encourage your child to use the restroom when he first wakes up, before meals, before bedtime, and soon before leaving the house.

CHAPTER 15

BONUS

41 MODERN PARENTING SOLUTIONS AND TIPS

POTTY TRAINING SUCCESSFULLY

Keep a constant check on your child at first, otherwise, he will go everywhere.

Potty training a child who is already quite simple with the correct techniques and attitude. The most important suggestion is to make it fun for the child and not to make a big deal out of it. Make a big fuss about it when your youngster successfully uses the toilet, whether it's the first time or the twentieth. Give him a prize, but it doesn't have to be something physical - it can be a lot of clapping, leaping up and down, or a lot of praying.

Kids will typically do whatever it takes to make their mother happy, but they will also do whatever it takes to elicit a strong reaction from their parents. If they have an accident, then

If parents make a big fuss about it, it will happen again and again.

However, if the accident is ignored, no attention is paid to it, and no mention is made of it at all, it becomes a painful memory and is unlikely to occur more frequently than successful toilet excursions.

Another good tip is to stop using diapers and don't even start using other sorts of disposable training pants. Instead, move directly to clothes training pants, preferably with a favorite cartoon character, because they don't want to defecate or pee on their favorite cartoon character.

Create a reward system that allows your youngster to earn a treat or a badge of some sort when he successfully "accomplishes his mission." Chocolate always seems to be a well-received incentive; however, some parents may prefer offering ticklers and little toys or using a chart.

Remember that your child's first memory will be that he has learned to associate the soiled diaper with the potty.

He may express to you that he needs to use the restroom after he has already used his diaper. This is a critical first step!

Make potty training a simple game. Indulge his budding interest in music, football, or basketball by using a musical or sports-themed toilet paper. There are some great devices available that are designed to make toilet training entertaining, such as the Flash and Cher Potty Chair.

Continue the game to sustain his attention as he grows older.

Allow your son to experience the innate manly pleasure of aiming at objects floating in the potty when he reaches the point when he has successfully gone pee. One or two cereal rings

Always make a handy target from a box of Cheering, and they won't clog up you're plumbing.

Consider the act of flushing the toilet to be a reward in and of itself.

This not only encourages your child to use the toilet but also reinforces the need to only flush when necessary. It is never too early to start taking precautions to avoid the misfortune of a plumber's expense if your son flushes something unsuitable down the toilet.

As he proceeds through the training process, your little guy should no longer sleep in a crib and should instead sleep in a toddler bed where he can climb out and use the potty as needed during naps and overnight.

Stop wearing disposable diapers or training pants.

These products are designed to make your youngster feel comfortable after he has oiled himself. This is exactly what you don't want during potty training. Instead, use cloth diapers or traditional plastic training pants to cover his "big boy underwear." The more uncomfortable he is when he forgets to use the toilet, the faster he will progress through the toilet-training stage.

Spend time with an older child or another toddler who is already toilet trained and can encourage him to "be a big boy" by using the toilet. Peer learning and mentoring are extremely successful methods for potty training boys.

Allow your child to "pee on a tree" like his father or older brother when they are outside. Few things may make a little boy feel more manly than this, and he will enjoy the fiction of knowing he can do this instead of using his diaper or pull-up.

To get your child to stay still long enough to "do number two," sit next to him and read him a potty-training book. Many books have been published specifically for this purpose, and children adore them.

Take your youngster to the store and let them choose their potty chair.

Encourage him to decorate it with stickers and doodles to make it feel more like his.

Begin by simply allowing him to use it whenever he wants, for whatever reason. He may want to read a book while sitting on his potty, and he may also want to use the potty while wearing his diaper.

Simply sitting on it will make him feel more at ease.

Make potty time a habit. Set specific times for your child to sit on the potty for a few minutes; whether or not they use it doesn't matter.

Whether they exhibit signs of the need to go outside of the designated time, rush them to the potty chair and reward them if they successfully use the chair.

When they have accident, try NOT to get made. This process requires time and practice, and children should be rewarded for success rather than penalized for failure.

When your child has a "poo-poo" in their diaper, assist them in going to the bathroom. That will show them where the "poo-poo" is.

It will take some time. Potty training a boy can take several months on average, so don't rush and be patient.

Do not yell. Face reality and accept that accidents will occur on your journey. Don't yell or belittle him since it will send everything backward.

Take a shot. Sometimes persuading a lad to aim into the toilet \Properly can be a struggle in itself.

Should you stand or sit? Some parents start their children sitting down to pee, so the overall process is less confusing for them.

Allow Him to watch Dad. Kids learn by watching, so don't be afraid to let your toddler watch Dad or an older brother use the toilet.

Remove your shorts Make sure to put clothing on boys that are easy to remove when they are toilet training.

Be patient. One way to make the entire process easier is to adopt a relaxed attitude toward it and realize that training may take a long time.

Reminders. Little kids need to pee frequently, so make sure to wake them up at least every 30 minutes if they need to go.

Be open-minded and adaptable. It is easy to become confused with the abundance of (sometimes contradictory) potty training information available. Trying to decide which strategy is the best is not always straightforward.

Timing. Experts believe that if you start a child's potty training at the age of two, they will have control by the age of three.

Allow your toddler to take the lead. Do not impose toilet training on your child.

Some Practical Advice. If you live in a two-story house, buy two identical potties to avoid the crie of "I want the other potty" and subsequent toilet training mishaps as your little one sprints to the favorite potty chair.

Book and video Take the time to incorporate a few potty-training tale books into your toddler's reading time well before you want to begin training.

Chart and reward Be creative when deciding on the reward system you will use to motivate your toddler toward toileting independence.

Targets for toilets Fill the toilet bowl with Cheerios or a ping-pong ball for the little boys to shoot at.

Take them underwear shopping. Most children find it very exciting to be able to choose their own "real" underpants.

Teddy bear or toy Put a little Diaper on an old toy or teddy bear so your youngster has a friend to go through the training with.

Decorate the toilet. Allow your son to customize his potty using stickers. He will be eager to use it since he is so proud of it.

Help the team. Ensure that your friends and family are aware that toilet training is taking place.ss

Make the bathroom welcoming. Bathrooms are typically functional (in the absence of necessity). Put a few small toys and books in there to keep your son occupied while he is sitting on the potty.

Fun food. Constipation is a common problem for children who are learning to use the toilet. Ensure that their diet has been changed so that constipation-promoting foods (particularly processed foods) are limited. You may need to introduce new foods, such as fresh fruits and vegetables. Make them more enticing by cutting them into creative shapes with a knife or cookie cutter.

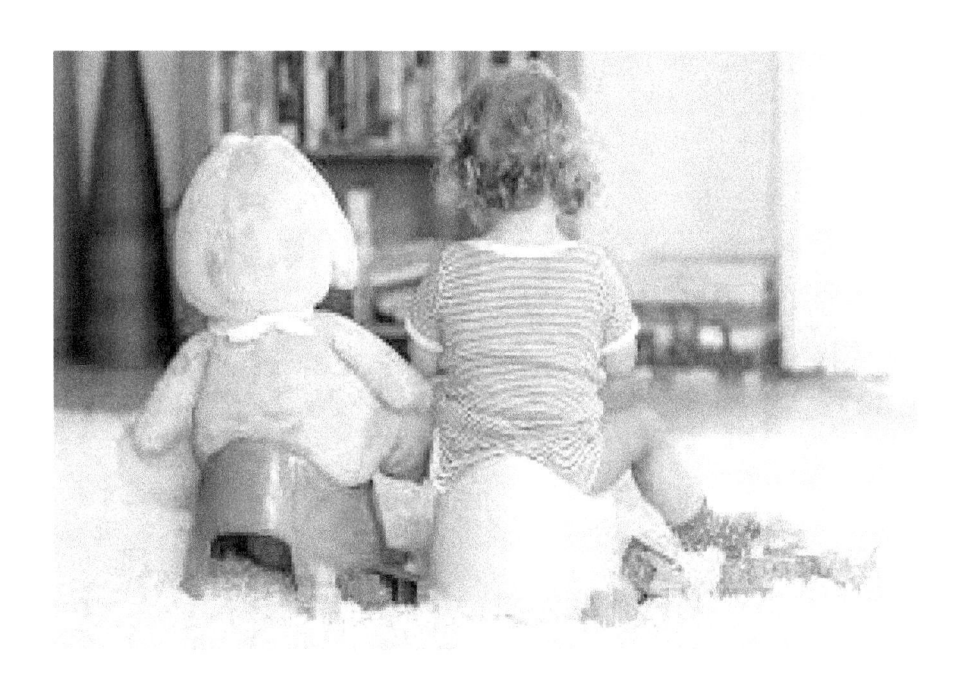

CPSIA information can be obtained
at www.ICGtesting.com
Printed in the USA
BVHW031504111022
649159BV00013B/1085

9 783986 537043